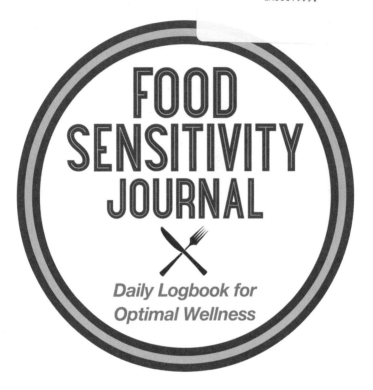

FOOD SENSITIVITY JOURNAL

Daily Logbook for Optimal Wellness

Molly Brennand

PETER PAUPER PRESS, INC.
WHITE PLAINS, NEW YORK

PETER PAUPER PRESS
Fine Books and Gifts Since 1928

Our Company

In 1928, at the age of twenty-two, Peter Beilenson began printing books on a small press in the basement of his parents' home in Larchmont, New York. Peter—and later, his wife, Edna—sought to create fine books that sold at "prices even a pauper could afford."

Today, still family owned and operated, Peter Pauper Press continues to honor our founders' legacy—and our customers' expectations—of beauty, quality, and value.

Designed by Margaret Rubiano
Images used under license from Shutterstock.com

Copyright © 2018
Peter Pauper Press, Inc.
202 Mamaroneck Avenue
White Plains, NY 10601
ISBN 978-1-4413-2772-7
Printed in Vietnam
7

Visit us at www.peterpauper.com

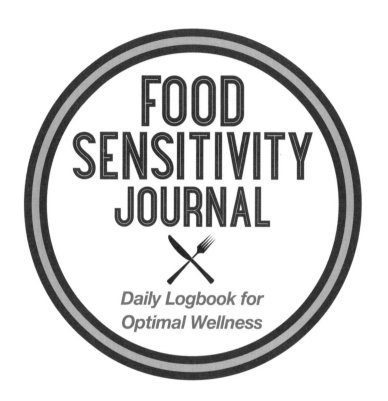

FOOD SENSITIVITY JOURNAL

Daily Logbook for
Optimal Wellness

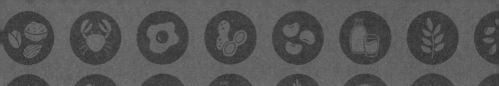

CONTENTS

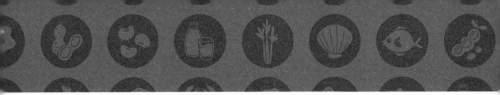

INTRODUCTION

- Do you ever wonder if there is a connection between that incessant need to clear your throat and a certain food you are eating?

- What about those peculiar little bumps on the back of your arms, the nagging pain in your left knee, or the eczema on your neck that just won't go away?

- Do fluctuating moods and energy levels seem to dictate your day without rhyme or reason?

- What about that back pain, those watery eyes, or the constipation, oh my!

It's entirely possible such vague and seemingly unrelated symptoms are closely linked to foods you eat. Research shows that food reactions, both immediate and delayed, are on the rise.

Keeping a food sensitivity journal provides you with a valuable tool that can help you identify foods that may be triggering physical and emotional discomfort. Beginning such a detailed approach to tracking patterns with food, mood, and physical symptoms is an empowering step on the path toward reclaiming and enhancing your health and well-being.

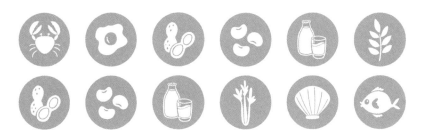

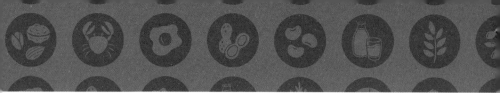

FOOD REACTIONS

If you are confused about the difference between **food allergies**, **sensitivities**, and **intolerances**, you are not alone. These phrases are often used interchangeably and because of this, are understood by many to have the same meaning. In fact, they are distinctly different. While these reactions are all responses to seemingly innocuous and benign foods, they are each handled differently by various aspects of the immune and the digestive systems. Let's take a closer look at these nuances to better understand how reactions to certain foods are addressed in the body.

FOOD ALLERGIES

A **food allergy** is the immune system's response to a perceived threat. When the immune system is taxed, it labels certain proteins from foods we ingest as dangerous. When a food is deemed a threat, the immune system will respond by calling in an elite unit of cells called **immunoglobulin E**, or **IgE**.

These produce an inflammatory response within the body and the signs and symptoms we typically associate with food allergies. These symptoms include, but are not limited to, breathing difficulties, swelling, hives, and vomiting. All usually occur within seconds or minutes of ingesting the offending food. These are all examples of an **IgE-mediated immune response**, with **anaphylactic shock** (a sudden and often life-threatening reaction) being the most severe.

FOOD SENSITIVITIES

A food sensitivity is also a response from the immune system, but one that generates a different type of immunoglobulin called **Immunoglobulin G**, or **IgG**. The distinguishing factor between these separate functions of the immune system lies in their response times. While an IgE response comes on fast and can be deadly, an IgG response is typically delayed and can produce a vague array of symptoms.

Common signs and symptoms of food sensitivities can include brain "fog," fatigue, eczema, bad breath, headaches, sleep issues, muscle and/or joint pain, digestive distress such as gas and bloating, asthma, acne, depression, anxiety, hyperactivity, and chronic rhinitis.

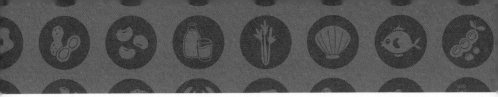

While it is not uncommon to see overlapping signs and symptoms with a food allergy, it is important to remember that a food allergy will deliver its message sooner rather than later, while a food sensitivity will always be late to the party.

FOOD INTOLERANCES

A **food intolerance** does not directly involve the immune system; the signs and symptoms will typically manifest within the confines of the **digestive system**. To explain this concept, let's focus on the reactions experienced by some of us after we consume dairy products.

If an individual is reacting to a **protein in milk** (such as **casein**) with a set of symptoms we typically interpret as an allergy, this would normally be considered an **IgE immune-mediated** allergic response.

But, if an individual has problems digesting the type of **milk sugar** called **lactose**, and therefore is having difficulty breaking down the lactose, an inflammatory state within the digestive tract will take hold, creating the perfect environment for diarrhea and abdominal cramping. This is more likely to be an example of **lactose intolerance** occurring within the digestive system. The immune system would not be involved in this case.

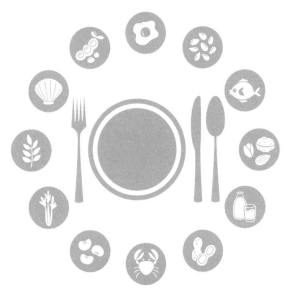

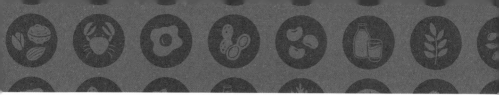

INSTRUCTIONS FOR USING THIS JOURNAL

Now that we have covered some of the basics with regard to types of food reactions, it's time to start tracking. There are enough log pages within this journal for you to track your meals, snacks, mood, and more for two months.

Keeping a daily log of what you eat and how you feel will ultimately cultivate a greater sense of awareness of the subtleties of how food affects you. With a little detective work, you will be on your way to achieving the vibrant health you want.

The **Daily Log Pages** within this journal include several sections that will not only help you capture the information you need to determine which foods might be derailing your health, but will also help you to identify lifestyle habits that might in turn influence your food choices.

While you are filling out the journal, commit yourself to gathering data without making judgments or assumptions. Making connections between your overall well-being and problematic foods will come at the end, once you have completed your journal. You are encouraged to dive in with an open and curious mind. The result will hopefully culminate in a greater awareness of and appreciation for your health and well-being. As you read through the instructions, please refer to the pre-filled sample log page (on pages 18 and 19) for reference.

MEALS/SNACKS AND LOCATIONS

On the **Daily Log Pages**, you'll find designated areas in which to record the standard three meals a day, along with two additional areas to record snacks. This is also the place to record any beverages you consume **other than water**. There is a separate area for recording hydration—please reserve that section for water only.

Locations: Within the designated meal and snack areas, you will notice a section to record the location where you eat and the time when you eat. Eating breakfast at the kitchen table will impact digestion differently than inhaling a donut on the subway on the way to work. Making note of the location will later help you determine whether the jolting subway ride caused your upset stomach or whether the suspicious ingredients

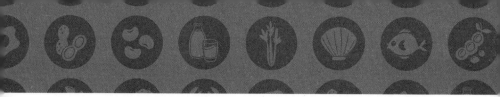

in the donut ultimately contributed to your gas and bloating. Enjoying a shrimp salad at a restaurant might produce a set of signs and symptoms that wouldn't normally arise when you make a shrimp salad in your own kitchen. Where we eat our meals and how we eat them can impact our health significantly.

Times: Writing down when you eat, and the time when signs and symptoms manifest can certainly be helpful in determining food allergies versus food sensitivities. If you have a food allergy, however, you are probably already aware of it based on your reaction time. Recording the time can help you better understand hunger and satiety signals, and can also help you become more aware of blood sugar imbalances that could be contributing to "hangry" or lethargic feelings throughout the day.

MOODS/SIGNS/SYMPTOMS/REACTIONS

There can be a tendency to match feelings with the meal you are eating. If you are experiencing a sense of calm or are feeling anxious, rushed, or have heartburn while eating, then make a note of it. That is relevant.

However, an important aspect of keeping a food sensitivity journal is keeping track of all moods, signs, and/or symptoms throughout the day, regardless of when they happen— not just when you are eating. Reserve this section for any emotional or psychological states that may arise during the day as well as physical signs and symptoms you experience. Be sure to record the time.

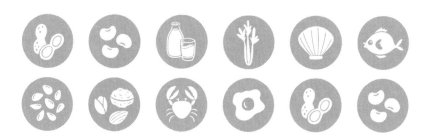

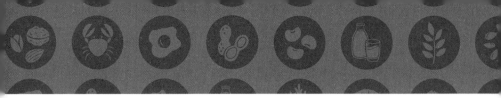

BOWEL MOVEMENTS

If you are wincing at the thought of having to observe and record your bowel movements, consider this: Taking a few seconds to peer into the bowl after the deed is done is the best (and cheapest) diagnostic tool you have for assessing your body's internal landscape and current expression of health.

For you shy folks, you can refer to the **Bristol Stool Chart** on the next page for poop descriptions. Simply record the designated number that best describes your bowel movement. For example, the Bristol Stool Chart classifies normal, healthy bowel movements as type 3 or 4. Types 1 and 2 are identified with constipation, while types 5, 6, and 7 are classified as various states of diarrhea. Pick the number that best describes your poop. Don't forget to note the time of elimination—this can be useful in determining which foods might be contributing to loose stools, constipation, and/or diarrhea.
Are you running to the bathroom like clockwork an hour after your triple latte with foam? Or does it take a week before you notice evidence of a beet salad in the toilet? Do your stools often float? Does the smell linger long after you wave bye-bye? Do you see undigested food particles in the bowl? These are all clues that your digestive system is under duress.

Tracking the food that's going in and paying attention to the poop that is going out can make for some powerful discoveries.

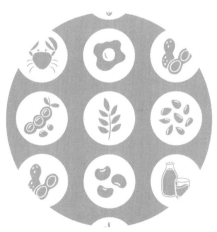

Bristol Stool Chart

Type 1		Separate hard lumps, like nuts (hard to pass)
Type 2		Sausage-shaped but lumpy
Type 3		Like a sausage but with cracks on the surface
Type 4		Like a sausage or snake, smooth and soft
Type 5		Soft blobs with clear-cut edges
Type 6		Fluffy pieces with ragged edges, a mushy stool
Type 7		Watery, no solid pieces, entirely liquid

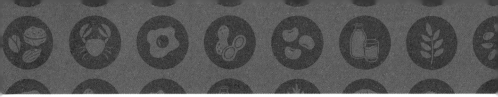

HYDRATION

Are you reaping the benefits of drinking enough water every day? Sometimes our body will seem to signal that we are hungry, when in fact we are thirsty. Tracking your daily water intake can be the most eye-opening aspect of the food log. Most likely you will discover you are not drinking enough water each day. Water aids the body in flushing out toxins via the urine and bowels. If you have a tendency toward constipation, drinking more water can help. In the hydration section, simply cross out or circle the amount of 8-ounce glasses of water you consume in a day. Most of us need to drink at least 7 glasses of water per day and many of us need to drink more.

SLEEP

Tracking your sleep for several days or weeks can give you great insight into how food choices may impact your sleep—as well as how your sleep might affect your food choices. What happens to your sleep when you cut out or cut down on caffeine, alcohol, sugar, or processed foods? If you don't get enough sleep, are you more inclined to drink a double espresso and eat a pastry to get your engine revving? Do certain foods promote an anxious or calm state in the body in the evening as your bedtime approaches? If you adjust your bedtime does it affect your quality of sleep and/or your wake time? These are all examples of questions that would most likely be answered after tracking your sleep hygiene and routine for an extended period.

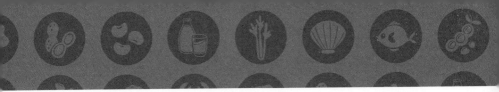

MEDICATIONS/VITAMINS/SUPPLEMENTS

If you are currently taking or beginning to take any new supplements and/or medications while you are filling out the journal, be sure to make a note and track how your body feels on the products. Record the day you started taking the medications or vitamins, doses, the time of day you take them, and any new signs and symptoms that emerge.

There can be adverse side effects to both medications and vitamins and they can also have hidden fillers and various binding agents that can cause myriad reactions. For example, fish oil supplements often contain vitamin E in the form of "mixed tocopherols." The vitamin E which provides antioxidants to help preserve the fish oil is sometimes sourced from soybeans. Many people today are either allergic or sensitive to soy and this is just one example of how you might be taking fish oil for all the right reasons but it might be doing more harm than good.

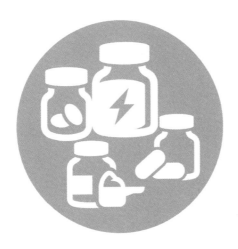

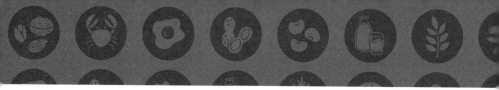

NOW WHAT?

If you have successfully completed your journal, congratulations are in order! Hopefully, you were able to gain some insight regarding your current state of health. You have successfully mastered the first step in identifying problem foods. The question at this point in the process is "Now what?" If you are still ingesting these newly identified problem foods daily, your body most likely needs a break from them to heal.

An appropriate next step would be implementing a trial elimination diet under the guidance and support of an experienced health care professional. Seeking out an individual who recognizes the value in distinguishing the difference between the various types of food reactions you are experiencing is important. A functional nutritionist and/or functional medical doctor can work with you to further support your efforts and help you get to the root cause of your health issues.

This journal will undoubtedly serve as a gold mine of pertinent information for the lucky practitioner who may become part of your health care team or for the practitioner you might be working with exclusively. Either way, you have taken the most important step of all and in doing so, you have made an invaluable investment in yourself.

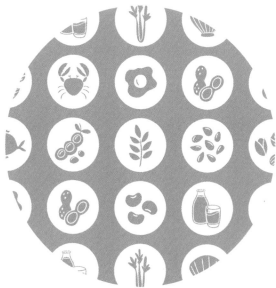

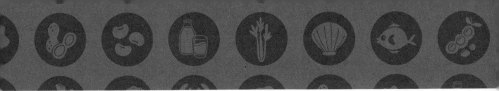

HELPFUL RESOURCES

Organizations

- The Functional Nutrition Alliance http://www.replenishpdx.com/counseling
- The Institute for Functional Medicine www.ifm.org
- Food Allergy Research & Education www.foodallergy.org
- BioSET www.bioset.net
- Nambudripad's Allergy Elimination Techniques (NAET) www.naet.com

Books

Is This Your Child? Discovering and Treating Unrecognized Allergies in Children and Adults. Rapp, Doris, M.D. New York: William Morrow & Co., 1991.

Allergic Girl: Adventures in Living Well with Food Allergies. Miller, Sloane. Hoboken, New Jersey: John Wiley & Sons, 2011.

Another Person's Poison: A History of Food Allergy. Smith, Matthew. New York: Columbia University Press, 2015.

The Allergy Solution: Unlock the Surprising, Hidden Truth about Why You Are Sick and How to Get Well. Galland, Leo, M.D., and Galland, Jonathan, J.D. Carlsbad, California: Hay House, Inc., 2016.

The Road to Immunity: How to Survive and Thrive in a Toxic World. Bock, Kenneth, M.D., and Sabin, Nellie. New York: Pocket Books, 1997.

The Complete Low-FODMAP Diet: A Revolutionary Plan for Managing IBS and Other Digestive Disorders. Shepherd, Sue, Ph.D., and Gibson, Peter, M.D. New York: The Experiment LLC, 2013.

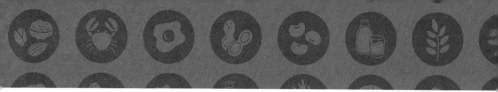

COMMON FOODS KNOWN TO CAUSE REACTIONS:

- Dairy
- Eggs
- Citrus
- Peanuts
- Shellfish
- Gluten
- Soy
- Corn
- Beef, lamb, and pork
- Coffee
- Foods high in FODMAPS*

*FODMAPS are defined as F.O.D.M.A.Ps: **f**ermentable **o**ligosaccharides, **d**isaccharides, **m**onosaccharides, **a**nd **p**olyols, and are a group of carbohydrates found in foods and some additives that do not absorb properly and that may cause digestive distress.

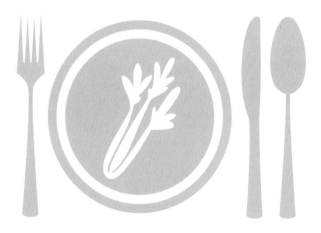

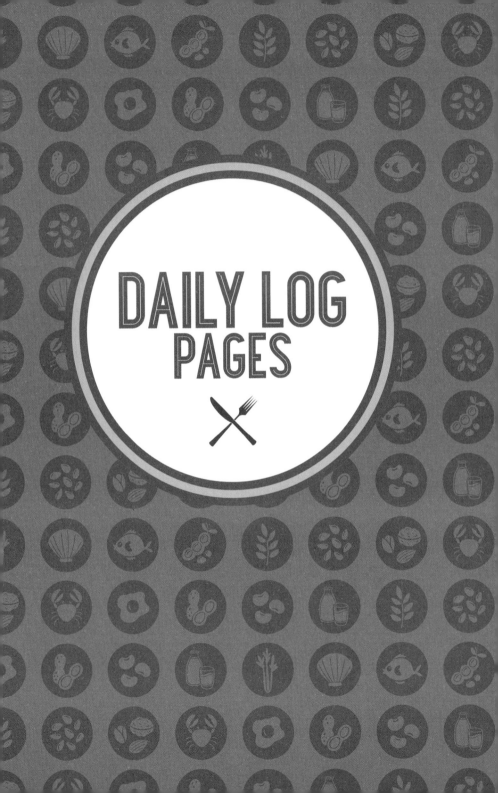

DAILY LOG
PAGES

SAMPLE LOG PAGES

DATE: _January 26_

MEAL 1 / LOCATION:	MOOD / SIGNS / SYMPTOMS / REACTIONS:
Breakfast at Lucy's Diner	Tired, hunger pains 8am
3 egg omelet with cheese,	Shaky and jittery by 9am
tomatoes, bacon	
1/2 cinnamon roll and 2 cups	
coffee w/ cream	
TIME: 9:15 a.m.	

BOWEL MOVEMENT TYPE (CIRCLE ONE): (1) 2 3 4 5 6 7

NOTES: Type 1, gray in color and hard. Lots of straining

TIME: 3:00 p.m.

MEAL 2 / LOCATION:	MOOD / SIGNS / SYMPTOMS / REACTIONS:
Lunch @ desk	Really tired and fatigued, hard to
Fish tacos w/ guacamole,	focus and irritable 2:45 p.m. to
salsa. Large coke and handful	around 4 p.m.
of corn chips	
TIME: 1:30 p.m.	

BOWEL MOVEMENT TYPE (CIRCLE ONE): 1 2 3 4 5 6 7

NOTES: none

TIME:

MEAL 3 / LOCATION:	MOOD / SIGNS / SYMPTOMS / REACTIONS:
Dinner out — French Bistro	Relaxed, calm, and peaceful
Steak frites, 2 glasses red wine,	during dinner
side salad and a few oysters	
	Super tired around 9 p.m. but
	second wind at 10 p.m.
TIME: 7:30 p.m.	

BOWEL MOVEMENT TYPE (CIRCLE ONE): 1 2 3 (4) 5 6 7

NOTES: Diarrhea at around 10:15 p.m. Lots of cramping and gas beforehand.

TIME: 10:15 p.m.

SAMPLE LOG PAGES

SNACK 1 / LOCATION / NOTES:

Power bar - at desk

	TIME: 11:00 a.m.

SNACK 2 / LOCATION / NOTES:

Ice coffee and chocolate chip cookie

coffee shop near work	TIME: 3:45 p.m.

LAST NIGHT'S SLEEP:

BEDTIME: 11 p.m.	WAKETIME: 6:00 a.m.

SLEEP QUALITY: Fell asleep fast but night waking 2x, hard to get up in the morning.

VITAMIN OR MEDICATION	REASON FOR TAKING	DOSAGE	DATE STARTED	COMMENTS/REACTIONS
Magnesium	sleep, digestion	500mg	1/26/2018	very helpful-sleep
		2 a day		better and more
				regular
B complex	mood, energy,	2/day	1/15/2018	2 a day, felt jittery.
	detox support			Better with one/day.

DAILY H2O INTAKE (CROSS OUT A DROP FOR EVERY GLASS CONSUMED)

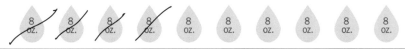

ADDITIONAL NOTES:

- I am noting better sleep quality on the days I stop eating by 7:30 p.m. and get in bed by 9:30 p.m.
- It seems that rice does not agree with me -- every time I eat it I experience gas and bloating within an hour after eating.
- I see that on the days I drink less than five glasses of water, it leads to constipation the next day

DATE: ....

MEAL 1 / LOCATION:	MOOD / SIGNS / SYMPTOMS / REACTIONS:

TIME:

BOWEL MOVEMENT TYPE (CIRCLE ONE):   1   2   3   4   5   6   7

NOTES:

	TIME:

MEAL 2 / LOCATION:	MOOD / SIGNS / SYMPTOMS / REACTIONS:

TIME:

BOWEL MOVEMENT TYPE (CIRCLE ONE):   1   2   3   4   5   6   7

NOTES:

	TIME:

MEAL 3 / LOCATION:	MOOD / SIGNS / SYMPTOMS / REACTIONS:

TIME:

BOWEL MOVEMENT TYPE (CIRCLE ONE):   1   2   3   4   5   6   7

NOTES:

	TIME:

SNACK 1 / LOCATION / NOTES:	
	TIME:
SNACK 2 / LOCATION / NOTES:	
	TIME:

LAST NIGHT'S SLEEP:

BEDTIME:	WAKETIME:

SLEEP QUALITY:

VITAMIN OR MEDICATION	REASON FOR TAKING	DOSAGE	DATE STARTED	COMMENTS/REACTIONS

DAILY H2O INTAKE (CROSS OUT A DROP FOR EVERY GLASS CONSUMED)

8 OZ. 8 OZ. 8 OZ. 8 OZ. 8 OZ. 8 OZ. 8 OZ. 8 OZ. 8 OZ. 8 OZ.

ADDITIONAL NOTES:

DATE: ....

MEAL 1 / LOCATION:	MOOD / SIGNS / SYMPTOMS / REACTIONS:
TIME:	

BOWEL MOVEMENT TYPE (CIRCLE ONE):   1   2   3   4   5   6   7

NOTES:

	TIME:

MEAL 2 / LOCATION:	MOOD / SIGNS / SYMPTOMS / REACTIONS:
TIME:	

BOWEL MOVEMENT TYPE (CIRCLE ONE):   1   2   3   4   5   6   7

NOTES:

	TIME:

MEAL 3 / LOCATION:	MOOD / SIGNS / SYMPTOMS / REACTIONS:
TIME:	

BOWEL MOVEMENT TYPE (CIRCLE ONE):   1   2   3   4   5   6   7

NOTES:

	TIME:

SNACK 1 / LOCATION / NOTES:	
	TIME:

SNACK 2 / LOCATION / NOTES:	
	TIME:

LAST NIGHT'S SLEEP:

BEDTIME:	WAKETIME:

SLEEP QUALITY:

VITAMIN OR MEDICATION	REASON FOR TAKING	DOSAGE	DATE STARTED	COMMENTS/REACTIONS

DAILY H2O INTAKE (CROSS OUT A DROP FOR EVERY GLASS CONSUMED)

8 OZ. 8 OZ. 8 OZ. 8 OZ. 8 OZ. 8 OZ. 8 OZ. 8 OZ. 8 OZ. 8 OZ.

ADDITIONAL NOTES:

DATE: ....

MEAL 1 / LOCATION:	MOOD / SIGNS / SYMPTOMS / REACTIONS:
TIME:	

BOWEL MOVEMENT TYPE (CIRCLE ONE):	1	2	3	4	5	6	7

NOTES:

	TIME:

MEAL 2 / LOCATION:	MOOD / SIGNS / SYMPTOMS / REACTIONS:
TIME:	

BOWEL MOVEMENT TYPE (CIRCLE ONE):	1	2	3	4	5	6	7

NOTES:

	TIME:

MEAL 3 / LOCATION:	MOOD / SIGNS / SYMPTOMS / REACTIONS:
TIME:	

BOWEL MOVEMENT TYPE (CIRCLE ONE):	1	2	3	4	5	6	7

NOTES:

	TIME:

SNACK 1 / LOCATION / NOTES:	
	TIME:
SNACK 2 / LOCATION / NOTES:	
	TIME:

LAST NIGHT'S SLEEP:	
BEDTIME:	WAKETIME:
SLEEP QUALITY:	

VITAMIN OR MEDICATION	REASON FOR TAKING	DOSAGE	DATE STARTED	COMMENTS/REACTIONS

DAILY H2O INTAKE (CROSS OUT A DROP FOR EVERY GLASS CONSUMED)

8 OZ. 8 OZ. 8 OZ. 8 OZ. 8 OZ. 8 OZ. 8 OZ. 8 OZ. 8 OZ. 8 OZ.

ADDITIONAL NOTES:

DATE: ....

MEAL 1 / LOCATION:	MOOD / SIGNS / SYMPTOMS / REACTIONS:
TIME:	

BOWEL MOVEMENT TYPE (CIRCLE ONE):   1   2   3   4   5   6   7

NOTES:

	TIME:

MEAL 2 / LOCATION:	MOOD / SIGNS / SYMPTOMS / REACTIONS:
TIME:	

BOWEL MOVEMENT TYPE (CIRCLE ONE):   1   2   3   4   5   6   7

NOTES:

	TIME:

MEAL 3 / LOCATION:	MOOD / SIGNS / SYMPTOMS / REACTIONS:
TIME:	

BOWEL MOVEMENT TYPE (CIRCLE ONE):   1   2   3   4   5   6   7

NOTES:

	TIME:

SNACK 1 / LOCATION / NOTES:	
	TIME:
SNACK 2 / LOCATION / NOTES:	
	TIME:

LAST NIGHT'S SLEEP:

BEDTIME:	WAKETIME:

SLEEP QUALITY:

VITAMIN OR MEDICATION	REASON FOR TAKING	DOSAGE	DATE STARTED	COMMENTS/REACTIONS

DAILY H2O INTAKE (CROSS OUT A DROP FOR EVERY GLASS CONSUMED)

8 OZ. 8 OZ. 8 OZ. 8 OZ. 8 OZ. 8 OZ. 8 OZ. 8 OZ. 8 OZ. 8 OZ.

ADDITIONAL NOTES:

DATE: ....

MEAL 1 / LOCATION:	MOOD / SIGNS / SYMPTOMS / REACTIONS:
TIME:	
BOWEL MOVEMENT TYPE (CIRCLE ONE): 1 2 3 4 5 6 7	
NOTES:	
	TIME:

MEAL 2 / LOCATION:	MOOD / SIGNS / SYMPTOMS / REACTIONS:
TIME:	
BOWEL MOVEMENT TYPE (CIRCLE ONE): 1 2 3 4 5 6 7	
NOTES:	
	TIME:

MEAL 3 / LOCATION:	MOOD / SIGNS / SYMPTOMS / REACTIONS:
TIME:	
BOWEL MOVEMENT TYPE (CIRCLE ONE): 1 2 3 4 5 6 7	
NOTES:	
	TIME:

SNACK 1 / LOCATION / NOTES:	
	TIME:

SNACK 2 / LOCATION / NOTES:	
	TIME:

LAST NIGHT'S SLEEP:	
BEDTIME:	WAKETIME:
SLEEP QUALITY:	

VITAMIN OR MEDICATION	REASON FOR TAKING	DOSAGE	DATE STARTED	COMMENTS/REACTIONS

DAILY H2O INTAKE (CROSS OUT A DROP FOR EVERY GLASS CONSUMED)

8 OZ.   8 OZ.   8 OZ.   8 OZ.   8 OZ.   8 OZ.   8 OZ.   8 OZ.   8 OZ.   8 OZ.

ADDITIONAL NOTES:

DATE: ....

MEAL 1 / LOCATION:	MOOD / SIGNS / SYMPTOMS / REACTIONS:
TIME:	

BOWEL MOVEMENT TYPE (CIRCLE ONE):   1   2   3   4   5   6   7

NOTES:

	TIME:

MEAL 2 / LOCATION:	MOOD / SIGNS / SYMPTOMS / REACTIONS:
TIME:	

BOWEL MOVEMENT TYPE (CIRCLE ONE):   1   2   3   4   5   6   7

NOTES:

	TIME:

MEAL 3 / LOCATION:	MOOD / SIGNS / SYMPTOMS / REACTIONS:
TIME:	

BOWEL MOVEMENT TYPE (CIRCLE ONE):   1   2   3   4   5   6   7

NOTES:

	TIME:

SNACK 1 / LOCATION / NOTES:	
	TIME:

SNACK 2 / LOCATION / NOTES:	
	TIME:

LAST NIGHT'S SLEEP:

BEDTIME:	WAKETIME:

SLEEP QUALITY:

VITAMIN OR MEDICATION	REASON FOR TAKING	DOSAGE	DATE STARTED	COMMENTS/REACTIONS

DAILY H2O INTAKE (CROSS OUT A DROP FOR EVERY GLASS CONSUMED)

8 OZ. 8 OZ. 8 OZ. 8 OZ. 8 OZ. 8 OZ. 8 OZ. 8 OZ. 8 OZ. 8 OZ.

ADDITIONAL NOTES:

DATE: ....

MEAL 1 / LOCATION:	MOOD / SIGNS / SYMPTOMS / REACTIONS:
TIME:	

BOWEL MOVEMENT TYPE (CIRCLE ONE):	1	2	3	4	5	6	7

NOTES:

	TIME:

MEAL 2 / LOCATION:	MOOD / SIGNS / SYMPTOMS / REACTIONS:
TIME:	

BOWEL MOVEMENT TYPE (CIRCLE ONE):	1	2	3	4	5	6	7

NOTES:

	TIME:

MEAL 3 / LOCATION:	MOOD / SIGNS / SYMPTOMS / REACTIONS:
TIME:	

BOWEL MOVEMENT TYPE (CIRCLE ONE):	1	2	3	4	5	6	7

NOTES:

	TIME:

SNACK 1 / LOCATION / NOTES:	
	TIME:

SNACK 2 / LOCATION / NOTES:	
	TIME:

LAST NIGHT'S SLEEP:

BEDTIME:	WAKETIME:

SLEEP QUALITY:

VITAMIN OR MEDICATION	REASON FOR TAKING	DOSAGE	DATE STARTED	COMMENTS/REACTIONS

DAILY H2O INTAKE (CROSS OUT A DROP FOR EVERY GLASS CONSUMED)

8 OZ.   8 OZ.   8 OZ.   8 OZ.   8 OZ.   8 OZ.   8 OZ.   8 OZ.   8 OZ.   8 OZ.

ADDITIONAL NOTES:

DATE: ....

MEAL 1 / LOCATION:	MOOD / SIGNS / SYMPTOMS / REACTIONS:
TIME:	

BOWEL MOVEMENT TYPE (CIRCLE ONE):	1	2	3	4	5	6	7

NOTES:

	TIME:

MEAL 2 / LOCATION:	MOOD / SIGNS / SYMPTOMS / REACTIONS:
TIME:	

BOWEL MOVEMENT TYPE (CIRCLE ONE):	1	2	3	4	5	6	7

NOTES:

	TIME:

MEAL 3 / LOCATION:	MOOD / SIGNS / SYMPTOMS / REACTIONS:
TIME:	

BOWEL MOVEMENT TYPE (CIRCLE ONE):	1	2	3	4	5	6	7

NOTES:

	TIME:

SNACK 1 / LOCATION / NOTES:	
	TIME:
SNACK 2 / LOCATION / NOTES:	
	TIME:

LAST NIGHT'S SLEEP:	
BEDTIME:	WAKETIME:
SLEEP QUALITY:	

VITAMIN OR MEDICATION	REASON FOR TAKING	DOSAGE	DATE STARTED	COMMENTS/REACTIONS

DAILY H2O INTAKE (CROSS OUT A DROP FOR EVERY GLASS CONSUMED)

8 OZ.   8 OZ.   8 OZ.   8 OZ.   8 OZ.   8 OZ.   8 OZ.   8 OZ.   8 OZ.   8 OZ.

ADDITIONAL NOTES:

DATE: ....

MEAL 1 / LOCATION:	MOOD / SIGNS / SYMPTOMS / REACTIONS:
TIME:	

BOWEL MOVEMENT TYPE (CIRCLE ONE):	1	2	3	4	5	6	7

NOTES:

	TIME:

MEAL 2 / LOCATION:	MOOD / SIGNS / SYMPTOMS / REACTIONS:
TIME:	

BOWEL MOVEMENT TYPE (CIRCLE ONE):	1	2	3	4	5	6	7

NOTES:

	TIME:

MEAL 3 / LOCATION:	MOOD / SIGNS / SYMPTOMS / REACTIONS:
TIME:	

BOWEL MOVEMENT TYPE (CIRCLE ONE):	1	2	3	4	5	6	7

NOTES:

	TIME:

SNACK 1 / LOCATION / NOTES:	
	TIME:
SNACK 2 / LOCATION / NOTES:	
	TIME:

LAST NIGHT'S SLEEP:	
BEDTIME:	WAKETIME:
SLEEP QUALITY:	

VITAMIN OR MEDICATION	REASON FOR TAKING	DOSAGE	DATE STARTED	COMMENTS/REACTIONS

DAILY H2O INTAKE (CROSS OUT A DROP FOR EVERY GLASS CONSUMED)

8 OZ.   8 OZ.   8 OZ.   8 OZ.   8 OZ.   8 OZ.   8 OZ.   8 OZ.   8 OZ.   8 OZ.

ADDITIONAL NOTES:

DATE: ....

MEAL 1 / LOCATION:	MOOD / SIGNS / SYMPTOMS / REACTIONS:
TIME:	

BOWEL MOVEMENT TYPE (CIRCLE ONE):	1	2	3	4	5	6	7

NOTES:

	TIME:

MEAL 2 / LOCATION:	MOOD / SIGNS / SYMPTOMS / REACTIONS:
TIME:	

BOWEL MOVEMENT TYPE (CIRCLE ONE):	1	2	3	4	5	6	7

NOTES:

	TIME:

MEAL 3 / LOCATION:	MOOD / SIGNS / SYMPTOMS / REACTIONS:
TIME:	

BOWEL MOVEMENT TYPE (CIRCLE ONE):	1	2	3	4	5	6	7

NOTES:

	TIME:

SNACK 1 / LOCATION / NOTES:	
	TIME:

SNACK 2 / LOCATION / NOTES:	
	TIME:

LAST NIGHT'S SLEEP:

BEDTIME:	WAKETIME:

SLEEP QUALITY:

VITAMIN OR MEDICATION	REASON FOR TAKING	DOSAGE	DATE STARTED	COMMENTS/REACTIONS

DAILY H2O INTAKE (CROSS OUT A DROP FOR EVERY GLASS CONSUMED)

8 OZ. 8 OZ. 8 OZ. 8 OZ. 8 OZ. 8 OZ. 8 OZ. 8 OZ. 8 OZ. 8 OZ.

ADDITIONAL NOTES:

DATE: ....

MEAL 1 / LOCATION:	MOOD / SIGNS / SYMPTOMS / REACTIONS:
TIME:	

BOWEL MOVEMENT TYPE (CIRCLE ONE):	1	2	3	4	5	6	7

NOTES:

	TIME:

MEAL 2 / LOCATION:	MOOD / SIGNS / SYMPTOMS / REACTIONS:
TIME:	

BOWEL MOVEMENT TYPE (CIRCLE ONE):	1	2	3	4	5	6	7

NOTES:

	TIME:

MEAL 3 / LOCATION:	MOOD / SIGNS / SYMPTOMS / REACTIONS:
TIME:	

BOWEL MOVEMENT TYPE (CIRCLE ONE):	1	2	3	4	5	6	7

NOTES:

	TIME:

SNACK 1 / LOCATION / NOTES:	
	TIME:

SNACK 2 / LOCATION / NOTES:	
	TIME:

LAST NIGHT'S SLEEP:

BEDTIME:	WAKETIME:

SLEEP QUALITY:

VITAMIN OR MEDICATION	REASON FOR TAKING	DOSAGE	DATE STARTED	COMMENTS/REACTIONS

DAILY H2O INTAKE (CROSS OUT A DROP FOR EVERY GLASS CONSUMED)

8 OZ.   8 OZ.   8 OZ.   8 OZ.   8 OZ.   8 OZ.   8 OZ.   8 OZ.   8 OZ.   8 OZ.

ADDITIONAL NOTES:

DATE: ....

MEAL 1 / LOCATION:	MOOD / SIGNS / SYMPTOMS / REACTIONS:
TIME:	

BOWEL MOVEMENT TYPE (CIRCLE ONE):	1	2	3	4	5	6	7

NOTES:

	TIME:

MEAL 2 / LOCATION:	MOOD / SIGNS / SYMPTOMS / REACTIONS:
TIME:	

BOWEL MOVEMENT TYPE (CIRCLE ONE):	1	2	3	4	5	6	7

NOTES:

	TIME:

MEAL 3 / LOCATION:	MOOD / SIGNS / SYMPTOMS / REACTIONS:
TIME:	

BOWEL MOVEMENT TYPE (CIRCLE ONE):	1	2	3	4	5	6	7

NOTES:

	TIME:

SNACK 1 / LOCATION / NOTES:	
	TIME:

SNACK 2 / LOCATION / NOTES:	
	TIME:

LAST NIGHT'S SLEEP:

BEDTIME:	WAKETIME:

SLEEP QUALITY:

VITAMIN OR MEDICATION	REASON FOR TAKING	DOSAGE	DATE STARTED	COMMENTS/REACTIONS

DAILY H2O INTAKE (CROSS OUT A DROP FOR EVERY GLASS CONSUMED)

8 OZ. 8 OZ. 8 OZ. 8 OZ. 8 OZ. 8 OZ. 8 OZ. 8 OZ. 8 OZ. 8 OZ.

ADDITIONAL NOTES:

DATE: ....

MEAL 1 / LOCATION:	MOOD / SIGNS / SYMPTOMS / REACTIONS:
TIME:	

| BOWEL MOVEMENT TYPE (CIRCLE ONE): 1 2 3 4 5 6 7 |

NOTES:
	TIME:

MEAL 2 / LOCATION:	MOOD / SIGNS / SYMPTOMS / REACTIONS:
TIME:	

| BOWEL MOVEMENT TYPE (CIRCLE ONE): 1 2 3 4 5 6 7 |

NOTES:
	TIME:

MEAL 3 / LOCATION:	MOOD / SIGNS / SYMPTOMS / REACTIONS:
TIME:	

| BOWEL MOVEMENT TYPE (CIRCLE ONE): 1 2 3 4 5 6 7 |

NOTES:
	TIME:

SNACK 1 / LOCATION / NOTES:	
	TIME:

SNACK 2 / LOCATION / NOTES:	
	TIME:

LAST NIGHT'S SLEEP:

BEDTIME:	WAKETIME:

SLEEP QUALITY:

VITAMIN OR MEDICATION	REASON FOR TAKING	DOSAGE	DATE STARTED	COMMENTS/REACTIONS

DAILY H2O INTAKE (CROSS OUT A DROP FOR EVERY GLASS CONSUMED)

8 OZ.	8 OZ.	8 OZ.	8 OZ.	8 OZ.	8 OZ.	8 OZ.	8 OZ.	8 OZ.	8 OZ.

ADDITIONAL NOTES:

DATE: ....

MEAL 1 / LOCATION:	MOOD / SIGNS / SYMPTOMS / REACTIONS:
TIME:	

BOWEL MOVEMENT TYPE (CIRCLE ONE): 1 2 3 4 5 6 7

NOTES:

	TIME:

MEAL 2 / LOCATION:	MOOD / SIGNS / SYMPTOMS / REACTIONS:
TIME:	

BOWEL MOVEMENT TYPE (CIRCLE ONE): 1 2 3 4 5 6 7

NOTES:

	TIME:

MEAL 3 / LOCATION:	MOOD / SIGNS / SYMPTOMS / REACTIONS:
TIME:	

BOWEL MOVEMENT TYPE (CIRCLE ONE): 1 2 3 4 5 6 7

NOTES:

	TIME:

SNACK 1 / LOCATION / NOTES:	
	TIME:

SNACK 2 / LOCATION / NOTES:	
	TIME:

LAST NIGHT'S SLEEP:

BEDTIME:	WAKETIME:

SLEEP QUALITY:

VITAMIN OR MEDICATION	REASON FOR TAKING	DOSAGE	DATE STARTED	COMMENTS/REACTIONS

DAILY H2O INTAKE (CROSS OUT A DROP FOR EVERY GLASS CONSUMED)

8 OZ.   8 OZ.   8 OZ.   8 OZ.   8 OZ.   8 OZ.   8 OZ.   8 OZ.   8 OZ.   8 OZ.

ADDITIONAL NOTES:

DATE: ....

MEAL 1 / LOCATION:	MOOD / SIGNS / SYMPTOMS / REACTIONS:
TIME:	

BOWEL MOVEMENT TYPE (CIRCLE ONE):   1   2   3   4   5   6   7

NOTES:

	TIME:

MEAL 2 / LOCATION:	MOOD / SIGNS / SYMPTOMS / REACTIONS:
TIME:	

BOWEL MOVEMENT TYPE (CIRCLE ONE):   1   2   3   4   5   6   7

NOTES:

	TIME:

MEAL 3 / LOCATION:	MOOD / SIGNS / SYMPTOMS / REACTIONS:
TIME:	

BOWEL MOVEMENT TYPE (CIRCLE ONE):   1   2   3   4   5   6   7

NOTES:

	TIME:

SNACK 1 / LOCATION / NOTES:

	TIME:

SNACK 2 / LOCATION / NOTES:

	TIME:

LAST NIGHT'S SLEEP:

BEDTIME:	WAKETIME:

SLEEP QUALITY:

VITAMIN OR MEDICATION	REASON FOR TAKING	DOSAGE	DATE STARTED	COMMENTS/REACTIONS

DAILY H2O INTAKE (CROSS OUT A DROP FOR EVERY GLASS CONSUMED)

8 OZ. 8 OZ. 8 OZ. 8 OZ. 8 OZ. 8 OZ. 8 OZ. 8 OZ. 8 OZ. 8 OZ.

ADDITIONAL NOTES:

DATE: ....

MEAL 1 / LOCATION:	MOOD / SIGNS / SYMPTOMS / REACTIONS:
TIME:	

BOWEL MOVEMENT TYPE (CIRCLE ONE):	1	2	3	4	5	6	7

NOTES:

	TIME:

MEAL 2 / LOCATION:	MOOD / SIGNS / SYMPTOMS / REACTIONS:
TIME:	

BOWEL MOVEMENT TYPE (CIRCLE ONE):	1	2	3	4	5	6	7

NOTES:

	TIME:

MEAL 3 / LOCATION:	MOOD / SIGNS / SYMPTOMS / REACTIONS:
TIME:	

BOWEL MOVEMENT TYPE (CIRCLE ONE):	1	2	3	4	5	6	7

NOTES:

	TIME:

SNACK 1 / LOCATION / NOTES:	
	TIME:

SNACK 2 / LOCATION / NOTES:	
	TIME:

LAST NIGHT'S SLEEP:

BEDTIME:	WAKETIME:

SLEEP QUALITY:

VITAMIN OR MEDICATION	REASON FOR TAKING	DOSAGE	DATE STARTED	COMMENTS/REACTIONS

DAILY H2O INTAKE (CROSS OUT A DROP FOR EVERY GLASS CONSUMED)

8 OZ.   8 OZ.   8 OZ.   8 OZ.   8 OZ.   8 OZ.   8 OZ.   8 OZ.   8 OZ.   8 OZ.

ADDITIONAL NOTES:

DATE: ....

MEAL 1 / LOCATION:	MOOD / SIGNS / SYMPTOMS / REACTIONS:
TIME:	

BOWEL MOVEMENT TYPE (CIRCLE ONE):   1   2   3   4   5   6   7

NOTES:

	TIME:

MEAL 2 / LOCATION:	MOOD / SIGNS / SYMPTOMS / REACTIONS:
TIME:	

BOWEL MOVEMENT TYPE (CIRCLE ONE):   1   2   3   4   5   6   7

NOTES:

	TIME:

MEAL 3 / LOCATION:	MOOD / SIGNS / SYMPTOMS / REACTIONS:
TIME:	

BOWEL MOVEMENT TYPE (CIRCLE ONE):   1   2   3   4   5   6   7

NOTES:

	TIME:

SNACK 1 / LOCATION / NOTES:	
	TIME:
SNACK 2 / LOCATION / NOTES:	
	TIME:

LAST NIGHT'S SLEEP:	
BEDTIME:	WAKETIME:
SLEEP QUALITY:	

VITAMIN OR MEDICATION	REASON FOR TAKING	DOSAGE	DATE STARTED	COMMENTS/REACTIONS

DAILY H2O INTAKE (CROSS OUT A DROP FOR EVERY GLASS CONSUMED)

8 OZ.   8 OZ.   8 OZ.   8 OZ.   8 OZ.   8 OZ.   8 OZ.   8 OZ.   8 OZ.   8 OZ.

ADDITIONAL NOTES:

DATE: ....

MEAL 1 / LOCATION:	MOOD / SIGNS / SYMPTOMS / REACTIONS:
TIME:	

BOWEL MOVEMENT TYPE (CIRCLE ONE):　　1　　2　　3　　4　　5　　6　　7

NOTES:

	TIME:

MEAL 2 / LOCATION:	MOOD / SIGNS / SYMPTOMS / REACTIONS:
TIME:	

BOWEL MOVEMENT TYPE (CIRCLE ONE):　　1　　2　　3　　4　　5　　6　　7

NOTES:

	TIME:

MEAL 3 / LOCATION:	MOOD / SIGNS / SYMPTOMS / REACTIONS:
TIME:	

BOWEL MOVEMENT TYPE (CIRCLE ONE):　　1　　2　　3　　4　　5　　6　　7

NOTES:

	TIME:

SNACK 1 / LOCATION / NOTES:	
	TIME:
SNACK 2 / LOCATION / NOTES:	
	TIME:

LAST NIGHT'S SLEEP:

BEDTIME:	WAKETIME:

SLEEP QUALITY:

VITAMIN OR MEDICATION	REASON FOR TAKING	DOSAGE	DATE STARTED	COMMENTS/REACTIONS

DAILY H2O INTAKE (CROSS OUT A DROP FOR EVERY GLASS CONSUMED)

8 OZ.   8 OZ.   8 OZ.   8 OZ.   8 OZ.   8 OZ.   8 OZ.   8 OZ.   8 OZ.   8 OZ.

ADDITIONAL NOTES:

DATE: ....

MEAL 1 / LOCATION:	MOOD / SIGNS / SYMPTOMS / REACTIONS:
TIME:	

BOWEL MOVEMENT TYPE (CIRCLE ONE):	1	2	3	4	5	6	7

NOTES:

	TIME:

MEAL 2 / LOCATION:	MOOD / SIGNS / SYMPTOMS / REACTIONS:
TIME:	

BOWEL MOVEMENT TYPE (CIRCLE ONE):	1	2	3	4	5	6	7

NOTES:

	TIME:

MEAL 3 / LOCATION:	MOOD / SIGNS / SYMPTOMS / REACTIONS:
TIME:	

BOWEL MOVEMENT TYPE (CIRCLE ONE):	1	2	3	4	5	6	7

NOTES:

	TIME:

SNACK 1 / LOCATION / NOTES:	
	TIME:

SNACK 2 / LOCATION / NOTES:	
	TIME:

LAST NIGHT'S SLEEP:

BEDTIME:	WAKETIME:

SLEEP QUALITY:

VITAMIN OR MEDICATION	REASON FOR TAKING	DOSAGE	DATE STARTED	COMMENTS/REACTIONS

DAILY H2O INTAKE (CROSS OUT A DROP FOR EVERY GLASS CONSUMED)

8 OZ. 8 OZ. 8 OZ. 8 OZ. 8 OZ. 8 OZ. 8 OZ. 8 OZ. 8 OZ. 8 OZ.

ADDITIONAL NOTES:

DATE: ....

MEAL 1 / LOCATION:	MOOD / SIGNS / SYMPTOMS / REACTIONS:
TIME:	

BOWEL MOVEMENT TYPE (CIRCLE ONE):　　1　　2　　3　　4　　5　　6　　7

NOTES:

	TIME:

MEAL 2 / LOCATION:	MOOD / SIGNS / SYMPTOMS / REACTIONS:
TIME:	

BOWEL MOVEMENT TYPE (CIRCLE ONE):　　1　　2　　3　　4　　5　　6　　7

NOTES:

	TIME:

MEAL 3 / LOCATION:	MOOD / SIGNS / SYMPTOMS / REACTIONS:
TIME:	

BOWEL MOVEMENT TYPE (CIRCLE ONE):　　1　　2　　3　　4　　5　　6　　7

NOTES:

	TIME:

SNACK 1 / LOCATION / NOTES:	
	TIME:
SNACK 2 / LOCATION / NOTES:	
	TIME:

LAST NIGHT'S SLEEP:	
BEDTIME:	WAKETIME:
SLEEP QUALITY:	

VITAMIN OR MEDICATION	REASON FOR TAKING	DOSAGE	DATE STARTED	COMMENTS/REACTIONS

DAILY H2O INTAKE (CROSS OUT A DROP FOR EVERY GLASS CONSUMED)

8 OZ. 8 OZ. 8 OZ. 8 OZ. 8 OZ. 8 OZ. 8 OZ. 8 OZ. 8 OZ. 8 OZ.

ADDITIONAL NOTES:

DATE: ....

MEAL 1 / LOCATION:	MOOD / SIGNS / SYMPTOMS / REACTIONS:
TIME:	

BOWEL MOVEMENT TYPE (CIRCLE ONE):   1   2   3   4   5   6   7

NOTES:

	TIME:

MEAL 2 / LOCATION:	MOOD / SIGNS / SYMPTOMS / REACTIONS:
TIME:	

BOWEL MOVEMENT TYPE (CIRCLE ONE):   1   2   3   4   5   6   7

NOTES:

	TIME:

MEAL 3 / LOCATION:	MOOD / SIGNS / SYMPTOMS / REACTIONS:
TIME:	

BOWEL MOVEMENT TYPE (CIRCLE ONE):   1   2   3   4   5   6   7

NOTES:

	TIME:

SNACK 1 / LOCATION / NOTES:	
	TIME:

SNACK 2 / LOCATION / NOTES:	
	TIME:

LAST NIGHT'S SLEEP:

BEDTIME:	WAKETIME:

SLEEP QUALITY:

VITAMIN OR MEDICATION	REASON FOR TAKING	DOSAGE	DATE STARTED	COMMENTS/REACTIONS

DAILY H2O INTAKE (CROSS OUT A DROP FOR EVERY GLASS CONSUMED)

8 OZ. 8 OZ. 8 OZ. 8 OZ. 8 OZ. 8 OZ. 8 OZ. 8 OZ. 8 OZ. 8 OZ.

ADDITIONAL NOTES:

DATE: ....

MEAL 1 / LOCATION:	MOOD / SIGNS / SYMPTOMS / REACTIONS:
TIME:	

BOWEL MOVEMENT TYPE (CIRCLE ONE):   1   2   3   4   5   6   7

NOTES:

	TIME:

MEAL 2 / LOCATION:	MOOD / SIGNS / SYMPTOMS / REACTIONS:
TIME:	

BOWEL MOVEMENT TYPE (CIRCLE ONE):   1   2   3   4   5   6   7

NOTES:

	TIME:

MEAL 3 / LOCATION:	MOOD / SIGNS / SYMPTOMS / REACTIONS:
TIME:	

BOWEL MOVEMENT TYPE (CIRCLE ONE):   1   2   3   4   5   6   7

NOTES:

	TIME:

SNACK 1 / LOCATION / NOTES:	
	TIME:
SNACK 2 / LOCATION / NOTES:	
	TIME:

LAST NIGHT'S SLEEP:

BEDTIME:	WAKETIME:

SLEEP QUALITY:

VITAMIN OR MEDICATION	REASON FOR TAKING	DOSAGE	DATE STARTED	COMMENTS/REACTIONS

DAILY H2O INTAKE (CROSS OUT A DROP FOR EVERY GLASS CONSUMED)

8 OZ. 8 OZ. 8 OZ. 8 OZ. 8 OZ. 8 OZ. 8 OZ. 8 OZ. 8 OZ. 8 OZ.

ADDITIONAL NOTES:

DATE: ....

MEAL 1 / LOCATION:	MOOD / SIGNS / SYMPTOMS / REACTIONS:
TIME:	
BOWEL MOVEMENT TYPE (CIRCLE ONE): 1 2 3 4 5 6 7	
NOTES:	
	TIME:

MEAL 2 / LOCATION:	MOOD / SIGNS / SYMPTOMS / REACTIONS:
TIME:	
BOWEL MOVEMENT TYPE (CIRCLE ONE): 1 2 3 4 5 6 7	
NOTES:	
	TIME:

MEAL 3 / LOCATION:	MOOD / SIGNS / SYMPTOMS / REACTIONS:
TIME:	
BOWEL MOVEMENT TYPE (CIRCLE ONE): 1 2 3 4 5 6 7	
NOTES:	
	TIME:

SNACK 1 / LOCATION / NOTES:	
	TIME:

SNACK 2 / LOCATION / NOTES:	
	TIME:

LAST NIGHT'S SLEEP:

BEDTIME:	WAKETIME:

SLEEP QUALITY:

VITAMIN OR MEDICATION	REASON FOR TAKING	DOSAGE	DATE STARTED	COMMENTS/REACTIONS

DAILY H2O INTAKE (CROSS OUT A DROP FOR EVERY GLASS CONSUMED)

8 OZ. 8 OZ. 8 OZ. 8 OZ. 8 OZ. 8 OZ. 8 OZ. 8 OZ. 8 OZ. 8 OZ.

ADDITIONAL NOTES:

DATE: ....

MEAL 1 / LOCATION:	MOOD / SIGNS / SYMPTOMS / REACTIONS:
TIME:	

BOWEL MOVEMENT TYPE (CIRCLE ONE):   1   2   3   4   5   6   7

NOTES:

	TIME:

MEAL 2 / LOCATION:	MOOD / SIGNS / SYMPTOMS / REACTIONS:
TIME:	

BOWEL MOVEMENT TYPE (CIRCLE ONE):   1   2   3   4   5   6   7

NOTES:

	TIME:

MEAL 3 / LOCATION:	MOOD / SIGNS / SYMPTOMS / REACTIONS:
TIME:	

BOWEL MOVEMENT TYPE (CIRCLE ONE):   1   2   3   4   5   6   7

NOTES:

	TIME:

SNACK 1 / LOCATION / NOTES:	
	TIME:
SNACK 2 / LOCATION / NOTES:	
	TIME:

LAST NIGHT'S SLEEP:

BEDTIME:	WAKETIME:

SLEEP QUALITY:

VITAMIN OR MEDICATION	REASON FOR TAKING	DOSAGE	DATE STARTED	COMMENTS/REACTIONS

DAILY H2O INTAKE (CROSS OUT A DROP FOR EVERY GLASS CONSUMED)

8 OZ.   8 OZ.   8 OZ.   8 OZ.   8 OZ.   8 OZ.   8 OZ.   8 OZ.   8 OZ.   8 OZ.

ADDITIONAL NOTES:

DATE: ....

MEAL 1 / LOCATION:	MOOD / SIGNS / SYMPTOMS / REACTIONS:
TIME:	

BOWEL MOVEMENT TYPE (CIRCLE ONE):   1   2   3   4   5   6   7

NOTES:

	TIME:

MEAL 2 / LOCATION:	MOOD / SIGNS / SYMPTOMS / REACTIONS:
TIME:	

BOWEL MOVEMENT TYPE (CIRCLE ONE):   1   2   3   4   5   6   7

NOTES:

	TIME:

MEAL 3 / LOCATION:	MOOD / SIGNS / SYMPTOMS / REACTIONS:
TIME:	

BOWEL MOVEMENT TYPE (CIRCLE ONE):   1   2   3   4   5   6   7

NOTES:

	TIME:

SNACK 1 / LOCATION / NOTES:	
	TIME:

SNACK 2 / LOCATION / NOTES:	
	TIME:

LAST NIGHT'S SLEEP:

BEDTIME:	WAKETIME:

SLEEP QUALITY:

VITAMIN OR MEDICATION	REASON FOR TAKING	DOSAGE	DATE STARTED	COMMENTS/REACTIONS

DAILY H2O INTAKE (CROSS OUT A DROP FOR EVERY GLASS CONSUMED)

8 OZ. 8 OZ. 8 OZ. 8 OZ. 8 OZ. 8 OZ. 8 OZ. 8 OZ. 8 OZ. 8 OZ.

ADDITIONAL NOTES:

DATE: ....

MEAL 1 / LOCATION:	MOOD / SIGNS / SYMPTOMS / REACTIONS:
TIME:	

BOWEL MOVEMENT TYPE (CIRCLE ONE):   1   2   3   4   5   6   7

NOTES:

	TIME:

MEAL 2 / LOCATION:	MOOD / SIGNS / SYMPTOMS / REACTIONS:
TIME:	

BOWEL MOVEMENT TYPE (CIRCLE ONE):   1   2   3   4   5   6   7

NOTES:

	TIME:

MEAL 3 / LOCATION:	MOOD / SIGNS / SYMPTOMS / REACTIONS:
TIME:	

BOWEL MOVEMENT TYPE (CIRCLE ONE):   1   2   3   4   5   6   7

NOTES:

	TIME:

SNACK 1 / LOCATION / NOTES:	
	TIME:

SNACK 2 / LOCATION / NOTES:	
	TIME:

LAST NIGHT'S SLEEP:

BEDTIME:	WAKETIME:

SLEEP QUALITY:

VITAMIN OR MEDICATION	REASON FOR TAKING	DOSAGE	DATE STARTED	COMMENTS/REACTIONS

DAILY H2O INTAKE (CROSS OUT A DROP FOR EVERY GLASS CONSUMED)

8 OZ. 8 OZ. 8 OZ. 8 OZ. 8 OZ. 8 OZ. 8 OZ. 8 OZ. 8 OZ. 8 OZ.

ADDITIONAL NOTES:

DATE: ....

MEAL 1 / LOCATION:	MOOD / SIGNS / SYMPTOMS / REACTIONS:
TIME:	

BOWEL MOVEMENT TYPE (CIRCLE ONE):   1   2   3   4   5   6   7

NOTES:

	TIME:

MEAL 2 / LOCATION:	MOOD / SIGNS / SYMPTOMS / REACTIONS:
TIME:	

BOWEL MOVEMENT TYPE (CIRCLE ONE):   1   2   3   4   5   6   7

NOTES:

	TIME:

MEAL 3 / LOCATION:	MOOD / SIGNS / SYMPTOMS / REACTIONS:
TIME:	

BOWEL MOVEMENT TYPE (CIRCLE ONE):   1   2   3   4   5   6   7

NOTES:

	TIME:

SNACK 1 / LOCATION / NOTES:	
	TIME:
SNACK 2 / LOCATION / NOTES:	
	TIME:

LAST NIGHT'S SLEEP:	
BEDTIME:	WAKETIME:
SLEEP QUALITY:	

VITAMIN OR MEDICATION	REASON FOR TAKING	DOSAGE	DATE STARTED	COMMENTS/REACTIONS

DAILY H2O INTAKE (CROSS OUT A DROP FOR EVERY GLASS CONSUMED)

8 OZ.   8 OZ.   8 OZ.   8 OZ.   8 OZ.   8 OZ.   8 OZ.   8 OZ.   8 OZ.   8 OZ.

ADDITIONAL NOTES:

DATE: ....

MEAL 1 / LOCATION:	MOOD / SIGNS / SYMPTOMS / REACTIONS:
TIME:	

BOWEL MOVEMENT TYPE (CIRCLE ONE):	1	2	3	4	5	6	7

NOTES:

	TIME:

MEAL 2 / LOCATION:	MOOD / SIGNS / SYMPTOMS / REACTIONS:
TIME:	

BOWEL MOVEMENT TYPE (CIRCLE ONE):	1	2	3	4	5	6	7

NOTES:

	TIME:

MEAL 3 / LOCATION:	MOOD / SIGNS / SYMPTOMS / REACTIONS:
TIME:	

BOWEL MOVEMENT TYPE (CIRCLE ONE):	1	2	3	4	5	6	7

NOTES:

	TIME:

SNACK 1 / LOCATION / NOTES:	
	TIME:

SNACK 2 / LOCATION / NOTES:	
	TIME:

LAST NIGHT'S SLEEP:

BEDTIME:	WAKETIME:

SLEEP QUALITY:

VITAMIN OR MEDICATION	REASON FOR TAKING	DOSAGE	DATE STARTED	COMMENTS/REACTIONS

DAILY H2O INTAKE (CROSS OUT A DROP FOR EVERY GLASS CONSUMED)

8 OZ. 8 OZ. 8 OZ. 8 OZ. 8 OZ. 8 OZ. 8 OZ. 8 OZ. 8 OZ. 8 OZ.

ADDITIONAL NOTES:

DATE: ....

MEAL 1 / LOCATION:	MOOD / SIGNS / SYMPTOMS / REACTIONS:
TIME:	

BOWEL MOVEMENT TYPE (CIRCLE ONE):	1	2	3	4	5	6	7

NOTES:

	TIME:

MEAL 2 / LOCATION:	MOOD / SIGNS / SYMPTOMS / REACTIONS:
TIME:	

BOWEL MOVEMENT TYPE (CIRCLE ONE):	1	2	3	4	5	6	7

NOTES:

	TIME:

MEAL 3 / LOCATION:	MOOD / SIGNS / SYMPTOMS / REACTIONS:
TIME:	

BOWEL MOVEMENT TYPE (CIRCLE ONE):	1	2	3	4	5	6	7

NOTES:

	TIME:

SNACK 1 / LOCATION / NOTES:	
	TIME:

SNACK 2 / LOCATION / NOTES:	
	TIME:

LAST NIGHT'S SLEEP:

BEDTIME:	WAKETIME:

SLEEP QUALITY:

VITAMIN OR MEDICATION	REASON FOR TAKING	DOSAGE	DATE STARTED	COMMENTS/REACTIONS

DAILY H2O INTAKE (CROSS OUT A DROP FOR EVERY GLASS CONSUMED)

8 OZ.   8 OZ.   8 OZ.   8 OZ.   8 OZ.   8 OZ.   8 OZ.   8 OZ.   8 OZ.   8 OZ.

ADDITIONAL NOTES:

DATE: ....

MEAL 1 / LOCATION:	MOOD / SIGNS / SYMPTOMS / REACTIONS:
TIME:	

BOWEL MOVEMENT TYPE (CIRCLE ONE):   1   2   3   4   5   6   7

NOTES:

	TIME:

MEAL 2 / LOCATION:	MOOD / SIGNS / SYMPTOMS / REACTIONS:
TIME:	

BOWEL MOVEMENT TYPE (CIRCLE ONE):   1   2   3   4   5   6   7

NOTES:

	TIME:

MEAL 3 / LOCATION:	MOOD / SIGNS / SYMPTOMS / REACTIONS:
TIME:	

BOWEL MOVEMENT TYPE (CIRCLE ONE):   1   2   3   4   5   6   7

NOTES:

	TIME:

SNACK 1 / LOCATION / NOTES:	
	TIME:

SNACK 2 / LOCATION / NOTES:	
	TIME:

LAST NIGHT'S SLEEP:

BEDTIME:	WAKETIME:

SLEEP QUALITY:

VITAMIN OR MEDICATION	REASON FOR TAKING	DOSAGE	DATE STARTED	COMMENTS/REACTIONS

DAILY H2O INTAKE (CROSS OUT A DROP FOR EVERY GLASS CONSUMED)

8 OZ. 8 OZ. 8 OZ. 8 OZ. 8 OZ. 8 OZ. 8 OZ. 8 OZ. 8 OZ. 8 OZ.

ADDITIONAL NOTES:

DATE: ....

MEAL 1 / LOCATION:	MOOD / SIGNS / SYMPTOMS / REACTIONS:
TIME:	

BOWEL MOVEMENT TYPE (CIRCLE ONE):   1   2   3   4   5   6   7

NOTES:

	TIME:

MEAL 2 / LOCATION:	MOOD / SIGNS / SYMPTOMS / REACTIONS:
TIME:	

BOWEL MOVEMENT TYPE (CIRCLE ONE):   1   2   3   4   5   6   7

NOTES:

	TIME:

MEAL 3 / LOCATION:	MOOD / SIGNS / SYMPTOMS / REACTIONS:
TIME:	

BOWEL MOVEMENT TYPE (CIRCLE ONE):   1   2   3   4   5   6   7

NOTES:

	TIME:

SNACK 1 / LOCATION / NOTES:	
	TIME:
SNACK 2 / LOCATION / NOTES:	
	TIME:

LAST NIGHT'S SLEEP:

BEDTIME:	WAKETIME:

SLEEP QUALITY:

VITAMIN OR MEDICATION	REASON FOR TAKING	DOSAGE	DATE STARTED	COMMENTS/REACTIONS

DAILY H2O INTAKE (CROSS OUT A DROP FOR EVERY GLASS CONSUMED)

8 OZ. 8 OZ. 8 OZ. 8 OZ. 8 OZ. 8 OZ. 8 OZ. 8 OZ. 8 OZ. 8 OZ.

ADDITIONAL NOTES:

DATE: ....

MEAL 1 / LOCATION:	MOOD / SIGNS / SYMPTOMS / REACTIONS:
TIME:	

BOWEL MOVEMENT TYPE (CIRCLE ONE):	1	2	3	4	5	6	7

NOTES:

	TIME:

MEAL 2 / LOCATION:	MOOD / SIGNS / SYMPTOMS / REACTIONS:
TIME:	

BOWEL MOVEMENT TYPE (CIRCLE ONE):	1	2	3	4	5	6	7

NOTES:

	TIME:

MEAL 3 / LOCATION:	MOOD / SIGNS / SYMPTOMS / REACTIONS:
TIME:	

BOWEL MOVEMENT TYPE (CIRCLE ONE):	1	2	3	4	5	6	7

NOTES:

	TIME:

SNACK 1 / LOCATION / NOTES:	
	TIME:
SNACK 2 / LOCATION / NOTES:	
	TIME:

LAST NIGHT'S SLEEP:

BEDTIME:	WAKETIME:

SLEEP QUALITY:

VITAMIN OR MEDICATION	REASON FOR TAKING	DOSAGE	DATE STARTED	COMMENTS/REACTIONS

DAILY H2O INTAKE (CROSS OUT A DROP FOR EVERY GLASS CONSUMED)

8 OZ. 8 OZ. 8 OZ. 8 OZ. 8 OZ. 8 OZ. 8 OZ. 8 OZ. 8 OZ. 8 OZ.

ADDITIONAL NOTES:

DATE: ....

MEAL 1 / LOCATION:	MOOD / SIGNS / SYMPTOMS / REACTIONS:
TIME:	

BOWEL MOVEMENT TYPE (CIRCLE ONE):   1   2   3   4   5   6   7

NOTES:

	TIME:

MEAL 2 / LOCATION:	MOOD / SIGNS / SYMPTOMS / REACTIONS:
TIME:	

BOWEL MOVEMENT TYPE (CIRCLE ONE):   1   2   3   4   5   6   7

NOTES:

	TIME:

MEAL 3 / LOCATION:	MOOD / SIGNS / SYMPTOMS / REACTIONS:
TIME:	

BOWEL MOVEMENT TYPE (CIRCLE ONE):   1   2   3   4   5   6   7

NOTES:

	TIME:

SNACK 1 / LOCATION / NOTES:

	TIME:

SNACK 2 / LOCATION / NOTES:

	TIME:

LAST NIGHT'S SLEEP:

BEDTIME:	WAKETIME:

SLEEP QUALITY:

VITAMIN OR MEDICATION	REASON FOR TAKING	DOSAGE	DATE STARTED	COMMENTS/REACTIONS

DAILY H2O INTAKE (CROSS OUT A DROP FOR EVERY GLASS CONSUMED)

8 OZ.   8 OZ.   8 OZ.   8 OZ.   8 OZ.   8 OZ.   8 OZ.   8 OZ.   8 OZ.   8 OZ.

ADDITIONAL NOTES:

DATE: ....

MEAL 1 / LOCATION:	MOOD / SIGNS / SYMPTOMS / REACTIONS:
TIME:	

BOWEL MOVEMENT TYPE (CIRCLE ONE):   1   2   3   4   5   6   7

NOTES:

	TIME:

MEAL 2 / LOCATION:	MOOD / SIGNS / SYMPTOMS / REACTIONS:
TIME:	

BOWEL MOVEMENT TYPE (CIRCLE ONE):   1   2   3   4   5   6   7

NOTES:

	TIME:

MEAL 3 / LOCATION:	MOOD / SIGNS / SYMPTOMS / REACTIONS:
TIME:	

BOWEL MOVEMENT TYPE (CIRCLE ONE):   1   2   3   4   5   6   7

NOTES:

	TIME:

SNACK 1 / LOCATION / NOTES:	
	TIME:

SNACK 2 / LOCATION / NOTES:	
	TIME:

LAST NIGHT'S SLEEP:

BEDTIME:	WAKETIME:

SLEEP QUALITY:

VITAMIN OR MEDICATION	REASON FOR TAKING	DOSAGE	DATE STARTED	COMMENTS/REACTIONS

DAILY H2O INTAKE (CROSS OUT A DROP FOR EVERY GLASS CONSUMED)

8 OZ. 8 OZ. 8 OZ. 8 OZ. 8 OZ. 8 OZ. 8 OZ. 8 OZ. 8 OZ. 8 OZ.

ADDITIONAL NOTES:

DATE: ....

MEAL 1 / LOCATION:	MOOD / SIGNS / SYMPTOMS / REACTIONS:
TIME:	

BOWEL MOVEMENT TYPE (CIRCLE ONE):   1   2   3   4   5   6   7

NOTES:

	TIME:

MEAL 2 / LOCATION:	MOOD / SIGNS / SYMPTOMS / REACTIONS:
TIME:	

BOWEL MOVEMENT TYPE (CIRCLE ONE):   1   2   3   4   5   6   7

NOTES:

	TIME:

MEAL 3 / LOCATION:	MOOD / SIGNS / SYMPTOMS / REACTIONS:
TIME:	

BOWEL MOVEMENT TYPE (CIRCLE ONE):   1   2   3   4   5   6   7

NOTES:

	TIME:

SNACK 1 / LOCATION / NOTES:	
	TIME:

SNACK 2 / LOCATION / NOTES:	
	TIME:

LAST NIGHT'S SLEEP:

BEDTIME:	WAKETIME:

SLEEP QUALITY:

VITAMIN OR MEDICATION	REASON FOR TAKING	DOSAGE	DATE STARTED	COMMENTS/REACTIONS

DAILY H2O INTAKE (CROSS OUT A DROP FOR EVERY GLASS CONSUMED)

8 OZ. 8 OZ. 8 OZ. 8 OZ. 8 OZ. 8 OZ. 8 OZ. 8 OZ. 8 OZ. 8 OZ.

ADDITIONAL NOTES:

DATE: ....

MEAL 1 / LOCATION:	MOOD / SIGNS / SYMPTOMS / REACTIONS:
TIME:	

BOWEL MOVEMENT TYPE (CIRCLE ONE):   1   2   3   4   5   6   7

NOTES:

	TIME:

MEAL 2 / LOCATION:	MOOD / SIGNS / SYMPTOMS / REACTIONS:
TIME:	

BOWEL MOVEMENT TYPE (CIRCLE ONE):   1   2   3   4   5   6   7

NOTES:

	TIME:

MEAL 3 / LOCATION:	MOOD / SIGNS / SYMPTOMS / REACTIONS:
TIME:	

BOWEL MOVEMENT TYPE (CIRCLE ONE):   1   2   3   4   5   6   7

NOTES:

	TIME:

SNACK 1 / LOCATION / NOTES:	
	TIME:
SNACK 2 / LOCATION / NOTES:	
	TIME:

LAST NIGHT'S SLEEP:

BEDTIME:	WAKETIME:

SLEEP QUALITY:

VITAMIN OR MEDICATION	REASON FOR TAKING	DOSAGE	DATE STARTED	COMMENTS/REACTIONS

DAILY H2O INTAKE (CROSS OUT A DROP FOR EVERY GLASS CONSUMED)

8 OZ. 8 OZ. 8 OZ. 8 OZ. 8 OZ. 8 OZ. 8 OZ. 8 OZ. 8 OZ. 8 OZ.

ADDITIONAL NOTES:

DATE: ....

MEAL 1 / LOCATION:	MOOD / SIGNS / SYMPTOMS / REACTIONS:
TIME:	

BOWEL MOVEMENT TYPE (CIRCLE ONE):	1	2	3	4	5	6	7

NOTES:

	TIME:

MEAL 2 / LOCATION:	MOOD / SIGNS / SYMPTOMS / REACTIONS:
TIME:	

BOWEL MOVEMENT TYPE (CIRCLE ONE):	1	2	3	4	5	6	7

NOTES:

	TIME:

MEAL 3 / LOCATION:	MOOD / SIGNS / SYMPTOMS / REACTIONS:
TIME:	

BOWEL MOVEMENT TYPE (CIRCLE ONE):	1	2	3	4	5	6	7

NOTES:

	TIME:

SNACK 1 / LOCATION / NOTES:	
	TIME:

SNACK 2 / LOCATION / NOTES:	
	TIME:

LAST NIGHT'S SLEEP:	
BEDTIME:	WAKETIME:
SLEEP QUALITY:	

VITAMIN OR MEDICATION	REASON FOR TAKING	DOSAGE	DATE STARTED	COMMENTS/REACTIONS

DAILY H2O INTAKE (CROSS OUT A DROP FOR EVERY GLASS CONSUMED)

8 OZ. 8 OZ. 8 OZ. 8 OZ. 8 OZ. 8 OZ. 8 OZ. 8 OZ. 8 OZ. 8 OZ.

ADDITIONAL NOTES:

DATE: ....

MEAL 1 / LOCATION:	MOOD / SIGNS / SYMPTOMS / REACTIONS:
TIME:	

BOWEL MOVEMENT TYPE (CIRCLE ONE):	1	2	3	4	5	6	7

NOTES:

	TIME:

MEAL 2 / LOCATION:	MOOD / SIGNS / SYMPTOMS / REACTIONS:
TIME:	

BOWEL MOVEMENT TYPE (CIRCLE ONE):	1	2	3	4	5	6	7

NOTES:

	TIME:

MEAL 3 / LOCATION:	MOOD / SIGNS / SYMPTOMS / REACTIONS:
TIME:	

BOWEL MOVEMENT TYPE (CIRCLE ONE):	1	2	3	4	5	6	7

NOTES:

	TIME:

SNACK 1 / LOCATION / NOTES:	
	TIME:

SNACK 2 / LOCATION / NOTES:	
	TIME:

LAST NIGHT'S SLEEP:

BEDTIME:	WAKETIME:

SLEEP QUALITY:

VITAMIN OR MEDICATION	REASON FOR TAKING	DOSAGE	DATE STARTED	COMMENTS/REACTIONS

DAILY H2O INTAKE (CROSS OUT A DROP FOR EVERY GLASS CONSUMED)

8 OZ. 8 OZ. 8 OZ. 8 OZ. 8 OZ. 8 OZ. 8 OZ. 8 OZ. 8 OZ. 8 OZ.

ADDITIONAL NOTES:

DATE: ....

MEAL 1 / LOCATION:	MOOD / SIGNS / SYMPTOMS / REACTIONS:
TIME:	

BOWEL MOVEMENT TYPE (CIRCLE ONE):	1	2	3	4	5	6	7

NOTES:

	TIME:

MEAL 2 / LOCATION:	MOOD / SIGNS / SYMPTOMS / REACTIONS:
TIME:	

BOWEL MOVEMENT TYPE (CIRCLE ONE):	1	2	3	4	5	6	7

NOTES:

	TIME:

MEAL 3 / LOCATION:	MOOD / SIGNS / SYMPTOMS / REACTIONS:
TIME:	

BOWEL MOVEMENT TYPE (CIRCLE ONE):	1	2	3	4	5	6	7

NOTES:

	TIME:

SNACK 1 / LOCATION / NOTES:	
	TIME:

SNACK 2 / LOCATION / NOTES:	
	TIME:

LAST NIGHT'S SLEEP:

BEDTIME:	WAKETIME:

SLEEP QUALITY:

VITAMIN OR MEDICATION	REASON FOR TAKING	DOSAGE	DATE STARTED	COMMENTS/REACTIONS

DAILY H2O INTAKE (CROSS OUT A DROP FOR EVERY GLASS CONSUMED)

8 OZ. 8 OZ. 8 OZ. 8 OZ. 8 OZ. 8 OZ. 8 OZ. 8 OZ. 8 OZ. 8 OZ.

ADDITIONAL NOTES:

DATE: ....

MEAL 1 / LOCATION:	MOOD / SIGNS / SYMPTOMS / REACTIONS:
TIME:	

BOWEL MOVEMENT TYPE (CIRCLE ONE):   1   2   3   4   5   6   7

NOTES:

	TIME:

MEAL 2 / LOCATION:	MOOD / SIGNS / SYMPTOMS / REACTIONS:
TIME:	

BOWEL MOVEMENT TYPE (CIRCLE ONE):   1   2   3   4   5   6   7

NOTES:

	TIME:

MEAL 3 / LOCATION:	MOOD / SIGNS / SYMPTOMS / REACTIONS:
TIME:	

BOWEL MOVEMENT TYPE (CIRCLE ONE):   1   2   3   4   5   6   7

NOTES:

	TIME:

SNACK 1 / LOCATION / NOTES:	
	TIME:

SNACK 2 / LOCATION / NOTES:	
	TIME:

LAST NIGHT'S SLEEP:

BEDTIME:	WAKETIME:

SLEEP QUALITY:

VITAMIN OR MEDICATION	REASON FOR TAKING	DOSAGE	DATE STARTED	COMMENTS/REACTIONS

DAILY H2O INTAKE (CROSS OUT A DROP FOR EVERY GLASS CONSUMED)

8 OZ. 8 OZ. 8 OZ. 8 OZ. 8 OZ. 8 OZ. 8 OZ. 8 OZ. 8 OZ. 8 OZ.

ADDITIONAL NOTES:

DATE: ....

MEAL 1 / LOCATION:	MOOD / SIGNS / SYMPTOMS / REACTIONS:
TIME:	

BOWEL MOVEMENT TYPE (CIRCLE ONE):	1	2	3	4	5	6	7

NOTES:	
	TIME:

MEAL 2 / LOCATION:	MOOD / SIGNS / SYMPTOMS / REACTIONS:
TIME:	

BOWEL MOVEMENT TYPE (CIRCLE ONE):	1	2	3	4	5	6	7

NOTES:	
	TIME:

MEAL 3 / LOCATION:	MOOD / SIGNS / SYMPTOMS / REACTIONS:
TIME:	

BOWEL MOVEMENT TYPE (CIRCLE ONE):	1	2	3	4	5	6	7

NOTES:	
	TIME:

SNACK 1 / LOCATION / NOTES:	
	TIME:
SNACK 2 / LOCATION / NOTES:	
	TIME:

LAST NIGHT'S SLEEP:

BEDTIME:	WAKETIME:

SLEEP QUALITY:

VITAMIN OR MEDICATION	REASON FOR TAKING	DOSAGE	DATE STARTED	COMMENTS/REACTIONS

DAILY H2O INTAKE (CROSS OUT A DROP FOR EVERY GLASS CONSUMED)

8 OZ.　8 OZ.　8 OZ.　8 OZ.　8 OZ.　8 OZ.　8 OZ.　8 OZ.　8 OZ.　8 OZ.

ADDITIONAL NOTES:

DATE: ....

MEAL 1 / LOCATION:	MOOD / SIGNS / SYMPTOMS / REACTIONS:
TIME:	

BOWEL MOVEMENT TYPE (CIRCLE ONE):   1   2   3   4   5   6   7

NOTES:

	TIME:

MEAL 2 / LOCATION:	MOOD / SIGNS / SYMPTOMS / REACTIONS:
TIME:	

BOWEL MOVEMENT TYPE (CIRCLE ONE):   1   2   3   4   5   6   7

NOTES:

	TIME:

MEAL 3 / LOCATION:	MOOD / SIGNS / SYMPTOMS / REACTIONS:
TIME:	

BOWEL MOVEMENT TYPE (CIRCLE ONE):   1   2   3   4   5   6   7

NOTES:

	TIME:

SNACK 1 / LOCATION / NOTES:	
	TIME:
SNACK 2 / LOCATION / NOTES:	
	TIME:

LAST NIGHT'S SLEEP:

BEDTIME:	WAKETIME:

SLEEP QUALITY:

VITAMIN OR MEDICATION	REASON FOR TAKING	DOSAGE	DATE STARTED	COMMENTS/REACTIONS

DAILY H2O INTAKE (CROSS OUT A DROP FOR EVERY GLASS CONSUMED)

8 OZ. 8 OZ. 8 OZ. 8 OZ. 8 OZ. 8 OZ. 8 OZ. 8 OZ. 8 OZ. 8 OZ.

ADDITIONAL NOTES:

DATE: ....

MEAL 1 / LOCATION:	MOOD / SIGNS / SYMPTOMS / REACTIONS:
TIME:	

BOWEL MOVEMENT TYPE (CIRCLE ONE):	1	2	3	4	5	6	7

NOTES:

	TIME:

MEAL 2 / LOCATION:	MOOD / SIGNS / SYMPTOMS / REACTIONS:
TIME:	

BOWEL MOVEMENT TYPE (CIRCLE ONE):	1	2	3	4	5	6	7

NOTES:

	TIME:

MEAL 3 / LOCATION:	MOOD / SIGNS / SYMPTOMS / REACTIONS:
TIME:	

BOWEL MOVEMENT TYPE (CIRCLE ONE):	1	2	3	4	5	6	7

NOTES:

	TIME:

SNACK 1 / LOCATION / NOTES:	
	TIME:

SNACK 2 / LOCATION / NOTES:	
	TIME:

LAST NIGHT'S SLEEP:

BEDTIME:	WAKETIME:

SLEEP QUALITY:

VITAMIN OR MEDICATION	REASON FOR TAKING	DOSAGE	DATE STARTED	COMMENTS/REACTIONS

DAILY H2O INTAKE (CROSS OUT A DROP FOR EVERY GLASS CONSUMED)

8 OZ.   8 OZ.   8 OZ.   8 OZ.   8 OZ.   8 OZ.   8 OZ.   8 OZ.   8 OZ.   8 OZ.

ADDITIONAL NOTES:

DATE: ....

MEAL 1 / LOCATION:

MOOD / SIGNS / SYMPTOMS / REACTIONS:

TIME:

BOWEL MOVEMENT TYPE (CIRCLE ONE):   1   2   3   4   5   6   7

NOTES:

TIME:

MEAL 2 / LOCATION:

MOOD / SIGNS / SYMPTOMS / REACTIONS:

TIME:

BOWEL MOVEMENT TYPE (CIRCLE ONE):   1   2   3   4   5   6   7

NOTES:

TIME:

MEAL 3 / LOCATION:

MOOD / SIGNS / SYMPTOMS / REACTIONS:

TIME:

BOWEL MOVEMENT TYPE (CIRCLE ONE):   1   2   3   4   5   6   7

NOTES:

TIME:

SNACK 1 / LOCATION / NOTES:	
	TIME:

SNACK 2 / LOCATION / NOTES:	
	TIME:

LAST NIGHT'S SLEEP:

BEDTIME:	WAKETIME:

SLEEP QUALITY:

VITAMIN OR MEDICATION	REASON FOR TAKING	DOSAGE	DATE STARTED	COMMENTS/REACTIONS

DAILY H2O INTAKE (CROSS OUT A DROP FOR EVERY GLASS CONSUMED)

8 OZ.   8 OZ.   8 OZ.   8 OZ.   8 OZ.   8 OZ.   8 OZ.   8 OZ.   8 OZ.   8 OZ.

ADDITIONAL NOTES:

DATE: ....

MEAL 1 / LOCATION:	MOOD / SIGNS / SYMPTOMS / REACTIONS:
TIME:	

BOWEL MOVEMENT TYPE (CIRCLE ONE):   1   2   3   4   5   6   7

NOTES:

	TIME:

MEAL 2 / LOCATION:	MOOD / SIGNS / SYMPTOMS / REACTIONS:
TIME:	

BOWEL MOVEMENT TYPE (CIRCLE ONE):   1   2   3   4   5   6   7

NOTES:

	TIME:

MEAL 3 / LOCATION:	MOOD / SIGNS / SYMPTOMS / REACTIONS:
TIME:	

BOWEL MOVEMENT TYPE (CIRCLE ONE):   1   2   3   4   5   6   7

NOTES:

	TIME:

SNACK 1 / LOCATION / NOTES:	
	TIME:

SNACK 2 / LOCATION / NOTES:	
	TIME:

LAST NIGHT'S SLEEP:

BEDTIME: **WAKETIME:**

SLEEP QUALITY:

VITAMIN OR MEDICATION	REASON FOR TAKING	DOSAGE	DATE STARTED	COMMENTS/REACTIONS

DAILY H2O INTAKE (CROSS OUT A DROP FOR EVERY GLASS CONSUMED)

8 OZ.   8 OZ.   8 OZ.   8 OZ.   8 OZ.   8 OZ.   8 OZ.   8 OZ.   8 OZ.   8 OZ.

ADDITIONAL NOTES:

DATE: ....

MEAL 1 / LOCATION:	MOOD / SIGNS / SYMPTOMS / REACTIONS:
TIME:	

BOWEL MOVEMENT TYPE (CIRCLE ONE):   1   2   3   4   5   6   7

NOTES:

	TIME:

MEAL 2 / LOCATION:	MOOD / SIGNS / SYMPTOMS / REACTIONS:
TIME:	

BOWEL MOVEMENT TYPE (CIRCLE ONE):   1   2   3   4   5   6   7

NOTES:

	TIME:

MEAL 3 / LOCATION:	MOOD / SIGNS / SYMPTOMS / REACTIONS:
TIME:	

BOWEL MOVEMENT TYPE (CIRCLE ONE):   1   2   3   4   5   6   7

NOTES:

	TIME:

SNACK 1 / LOCATION / NOTES:	
	TIME:

SNACK 2 / LOCATION / NOTES:	
	TIME:

LAST NIGHT'S SLEEP:

BEDTIME:	WAKETIME:

SLEEP QUALITY:

VITAMIN OR MEDICATION	REASON FOR TAKING	DOSAGE	DATE STARTED	COMMENTS/REACTIONS

DAILY H2O INTAKE (CROSS OUT A DROP FOR EVERY GLASS CONSUMED)

8 OZ.   8 OZ.   8 OZ.   8 OZ.   8 OZ.   8 OZ.   8 OZ.   8 OZ.   8 OZ.   8 OZ.

ADDITIONAL NOTES:

DATE: ....

MEAL 1 / LOCATION:	MOOD / SIGNS / SYMPTOMS / REACTIONS:
TIME:	

BOWEL MOVEMENT TYPE (CIRCLE ONE):   1   2   3   4   5   6   7

NOTES:

	TIME:

MEAL 2 / LOCATION:	MOOD / SIGNS / SYMPTOMS / REACTIONS:
TIME:	

BOWEL MOVEMENT TYPE (CIRCLE ONE):   1   2   3   4   5   6   7

NOTES:

	TIME:

MEAL 3 / LOCATION:	MOOD / SIGNS / SYMPTOMS / REACTIONS:
TIME:	

BOWEL MOVEMENT TYPE (CIRCLE ONE):   1   2   3   4   5   6   7

NOTES:

	TIME:

SNACK 1 / LOCATION / NOTES:	
	TIME:

SNACK 2 / LOCATION / NOTES:	
	TIME:

LAST NIGHT'S SLEEP:

BEDTIME:	WAKETIME:

SLEEP QUALITY:

VITAMIN OR MEDICATION	REASON FOR TAKING	DOSAGE	DATE STARTED	COMMENTS/REACTIONS

DAILY H2O INTAKE (CROSS OUT A DROP FOR EVERY GLASS CONSUMED)

8 OZ. · 8 OZ. · 8 OZ. · 8 OZ. · 8 OZ. · 8 OZ. · 8 OZ. · 8 OZ. · 8 OZ. · 8 OZ.

ADDITIONAL NOTES:

DATE: ....

MEAL 1 / LOCATION:	MOOD / SIGNS / SYMPTOMS / REACTIONS:
TIME:	

BOWEL MOVEMENT TYPE (CIRCLE ONE): 1 2 3 4 5 6 7

NOTES:

	TIME:

MEAL 2 / LOCATION:	MOOD / SIGNS / SYMPTOMS / REACTIONS:
TIME:	

BOWEL MOVEMENT TYPE (CIRCLE ONE): 1 2 3 4 5 6 7

NOTES:

	TIME:

MEAL 3 / LOCATION:	MOOD / SIGNS / SYMPTOMS / REACTIONS:
TIME:	

BOWEL MOVEMENT TYPE (CIRCLE ONE): 1 2 3 4 5 6 7

NOTES:

	TIME:

SNACK 1 / LOCATION / NOTES:	
	TIME:

SNACK 2 / LOCATION / NOTES:	
	TIME:

LAST NIGHT'S SLEEP:

BEDTIME:	WAKETIME:

SLEEP QUALITY:

VITAMIN OR MEDICATION	REASON FOR TAKING	DOSAGE	DATE STARTED	COMMENTS/REACTIONS

DAILY H2O INTAKE (CROSS OUT A DROP FOR EVERY GLASS CONSUMED)

8 OZ. 8 OZ. 8 OZ. 8 OZ. 8 OZ. 8 OZ. 8 OZ. 8 OZ. 8 OZ. 8 OZ.

ADDITIONAL NOTES:

DATE: ....

MEAL 1 / LOCATION:	MOOD / SIGNS / SYMPTOMS / REACTIONS:
TIME:	

BOWEL MOVEMENT TYPE (CIRCLE ONE):   1   2   3   4   5   6   7

NOTES:

	TIME:

MEAL 2 / LOCATION:	MOOD / SIGNS / SYMPTOMS / REACTIONS:
TIME:	

BOWEL MOVEMENT TYPE (CIRCLE ONE):   1   2   3   4   5   6   7

NOTES:

	TIME:

MEAL 3 / LOCATION:	MOOD / SIGNS / SYMPTOMS / REACTIONS:
TIME:	

BOWEL MOVEMENT TYPE (CIRCLE ONE):   1   2   3   4   5   6   7

NOTES:

	TIME:

SNACK 1 / LOCATION / NOTES:	
	TIME:
SNACK 2 / LOCATION / NOTES:	
	TIME:

LAST NIGHT'S SLEEP:

BEDTIME:	WAKETIME:

SLEEP QUALITY:

VITAMIN OR MEDICATION	REASON FOR TAKING	DOSAGE	DATE STARTED	COMMENTS/REACTIONS

DAILY H2O INTAKE (CROSS OUT A DROP FOR EVERY GLASS CONSUMED)

8 OZ.   8 OZ.   8 OZ.   8 OZ.   8 OZ.   8 OZ.   8 OZ.   8 OZ.   8 OZ.   8 OZ.

ADDITIONAL NOTES:

DATE: ....

MEAL 1 / LOCATION:	MOOD / SIGNS / SYMPTOMS / REACTIONS:
TIME:	

BOWEL MOVEMENT TYPE (CIRCLE ONE):   1   2   3   4   5   6   7

NOTES:

	TIME:

MEAL 2 / LOCATION:	MOOD / SIGNS / SYMPTOMS / REACTIONS:
TIME:	

BOWEL MOVEMENT TYPE (CIRCLE ONE):   1   2   3   4   5   6   7

NOTES:

	TIME:

MEAL 3 / LOCATION:	MOOD / SIGNS / SYMPTOMS / REACTIONS:
TIME:	

BOWEL MOVEMENT TYPE (CIRCLE ONE):   1   2   3   4   5   6   7

NOTES:

	TIME:

SNACK 1 / LOCATION / NOTES:	
	TIME:

SNACK 2 / LOCATION / NOTES:	
	TIME:

LAST NIGHT'S SLEEP:

BEDTIME:	WAKETIME:

SLEEP QUALITY:

VITAMIN OR MEDICATION	REASON FOR TAKING	DOSAGE	DATE STARTED	COMMENTS/REACTIONS

DAILY H2O INTAKE (CROSS OUT A DROP FOR EVERY GLASS CONSUMED)

8 OZ.   8 OZ.   8 OZ.   8 OZ.   8 OZ.   8 OZ.   8 OZ.   8 OZ.   8 OZ.   8 OZ.

ADDITIONAL NOTES:

DATE: ....

MEAL 1 / LOCATION:	MOOD / SIGNS / SYMPTOMS / REACTIONS:

TIME:

BOWEL MOVEMENT TYPE (CIRCLE ONE):   1   2   3   4   5   6   7

NOTES:

	TIME:

MEAL 2 / LOCATION:	MOOD / SIGNS / SYMPTOMS / REACTIONS:

TIME:

BOWEL MOVEMENT TYPE (CIRCLE ONE):   1   2   3   4   5   6   7

NOTES:

	TIME:

MEAL 3 / LOCATION:	MOOD / SIGNS / SYMPTOMS / REACTIONS:

TIME:

BOWEL MOVEMENT TYPE (CIRCLE ONE):   1   2   3   4   5   6   7

NOTES:

	TIME:

SNACK 1 / LOCATION / NOTES:	
	TIME:

SNACK 2 / LOCATION / NOTES:	
	TIME:

LAST NIGHT'S SLEEP:

BEDTIME:	WAKETIME:

SLEEP QUALITY:

VITAMIN OR MEDICATION	REASON FOR TAKING	DOSAGE	DATE STARTED	COMMENTS/REACTIONS

DAILY H2O INTAKE (CROSS OUT A DROP FOR EVERY GLASS CONSUMED)

8 OZ. 8 OZ. 8 OZ. 8 OZ. 8 OZ. 8 OZ. 8 OZ. 8 OZ. 8 OZ. 8 OZ.

ADDITIONAL NOTES:

DATE: ....

MEAL 1 / LOCATION:	MOOD / SIGNS / SYMPTOMS / REACTIONS:
TIME:	

BOWEL MOVEMENT TYPE (CIRCLE ONE):   1   2   3   4   5   6   7

NOTES:

	TIME:

MEAL 2 / LOCATION:	MOOD / SIGNS / SYMPTOMS / REACTIONS:
TIME:	

BOWEL MOVEMENT TYPE (CIRCLE ONE):   1   2   3   4   5   6   7

NOTES:

	TIME:

MEAL 3 / LOCATION:	MOOD / SIGNS / SYMPTOMS / REACTIONS:
TIME:	

BOWEL MOVEMENT TYPE (CIRCLE ONE):   1   2   3   4   5   6   7

NOTES:

	TIME:

SNACK 1 / LOCATION / NOTES:	
	TIME:

SNACK 2 / LOCATION / NOTES:	
	TIME:

LAST NIGHT'S SLEEP:	
BEDTIME:	WAKETIME:
SLEEP QUALITY:	

VITAMIN OR MEDICATION	REASON FOR TAKING	DOSAGE	DATE STARTED	COMMENTS/REACTIONS

DAILY H2O INTAKE (CROSS OUT A DROP FOR EVERY GLASS CONSUMED)

8 OZ. 8 OZ. 8 OZ. 8 OZ. 8 OZ. 8 OZ. 8 OZ. 8 OZ. 8 OZ. 8 OZ.

ADDITIONAL NOTES:

DATE: ....

MEAL 1 / LOCATION:	MOOD / SIGNS / SYMPTOMS / REACTIONS:
TIME:	

BOWEL MOVEMENT TYPE (CIRCLE ONE):   1   2   3   4   5   6   7

NOTES:

	TIME:

MEAL 2 / LOCATION:	MOOD / SIGNS / SYMPTOMS / REACTIONS:
TIME:	

BOWEL MOVEMENT TYPE (CIRCLE ONE):   1   2   3   4   5   6   7

NOTES:

	TIME:

MEAL 3 / LOCATION:	MOOD / SIGNS / SYMPTOMS / REACTIONS:
TIME:	

BOWEL MOVEMENT TYPE (CIRCLE ONE):   1   2   3   4   5   6   7

NOTES:

	TIME:

SNACK 1 / LOCATION / NOTES:

	TIME:

SNACK 2 / LOCATION / NOTES:

	TIME:

LAST NIGHT'S SLEEP:

BEDTIME:	WAKETIME:

SLEEP QUALITY:

VITAMIN OR MEDICATION	REASON FOR TAKING	DOSAGE	DATE STARTED	COMMENTS/REACTIONS

DAILY H2O INTAKE (CROSS OUT A DROP FOR EVERY GLASS CONSUMED)

8 OZ.   8 OZ.   8 OZ.   8 OZ.   8 OZ.   8 OZ.   8 OZ.   8 OZ.   8 OZ.   8 OZ.

ADDITIONAL NOTES:

DATE: ....

MEAL 1 / LOCATION:

MOOD / SIGNS / SYMPTOMS / REACTIONS:

TIME:

BOWEL MOVEMENT TYPE (CIRCLE ONE): 1 2 3 4 5 6 7

NOTES:

TIME:

MEAL 2 / LOCATION:

MOOD / SIGNS / SYMPTOMS / REACTIONS:

TIME:

BOWEL MOVEMENT TYPE (CIRCLE ONE): 1 2 3 4 5 6 7

NOTES:

TIME:

MEAL 3 / LOCATION:

MOOD / SIGNS / SYMPTOMS / REACTIONS:

TIME:

BOWEL MOVEMENT TYPE (CIRCLE ONE): 1 2 3 4 5 6 7

NOTES:

TIME:

SNACK 1 / LOCATION / NOTES:

	TIME:

SNACK 2 / LOCATION / NOTES:

	TIME:

LAST NIGHT'S SLEEP:

BEDTIME:	WAKETIME:

SLEEP QUALITY:

VITAMIN OR MEDICATION	REASON FOR TAKING	DOSAGE	DATE STARTED	COMMENTS/REACTIONS

DAILY H2O INTAKE (CROSS OUT A DROP FOR EVERY GLASS CONSUMED)

8 OZ.   8 OZ.   8 OZ.   8 OZ.   8 OZ.   8 OZ.   8 OZ.   8 OZ.   8 OZ.   8 OZ.

ADDITIONAL NOTES:

DATE: ....

MEAL 1 / LOCATION:	MOOD / SIGNS / SYMPTOMS / REACTIONS:
TIME:	

BOWEL MOVEMENT TYPE (CIRCLE ONE): 1   2   3   4   5   6   7

NOTES:

	TIME:

MEAL 2 / LOCATION:	MOOD / SIGNS / SYMPTOMS / REACTIONS:
TIME:	

BOWEL MOVEMENT TYPE (CIRCLE ONE): 1   2   3   4   5   6   7

NOTES:

	TIME:

MEAL 3 / LOCATION:	MOOD / SIGNS / SYMPTOMS / REACTIONS:
TIME:	

BOWEL MOVEMENT TYPE (CIRCLE ONE): 1   2   3   4   5   6   7

NOTES:

	TIME:

SNACK 1 / LOCATION / NOTES:	
	TIME:

SNACK 2 / LOCATION / NOTES:	
	TIME:

LAST NIGHT'S SLEEP:

BEDTIME:	WAKETIME:

SLEEP QUALITY:

VITAMIN OR MEDICATION	REASON FOR TAKING	DOSAGE	DATE STARTED	COMMENTS/REACTIONS

DAILY H2O INTAKE (CROSS OUT A DROP FOR EVERY GLASS CONSUMED)

8 OZ.   8 OZ.   8 OZ.   8 OZ.   8 OZ.   8 OZ.   8 OZ.   8 OZ.   8 OZ.   8 OZ.

ADDITIONAL NOTES:

DATE: ....

MEAL 1 / LOCATION:	MOOD / SIGNS / SYMPTOMS / REACTIONS:
TIME:	

BOWEL MOVEMENT TYPE (CIRCLE ONE):   1   2   3   4   5   6   7

NOTES:

	TIME:

MEAL 2 / LOCATION:	MOOD / SIGNS / SYMPTOMS / REACTIONS:
TIME:	

BOWEL MOVEMENT TYPE (CIRCLE ONE):   1   2   3   4   5   6   7

NOTES:

	TIME:

MEAL 3 / LOCATION:	MOOD / SIGNS / SYMPTOMS / REACTIONS:
TIME:	

BOWEL MOVEMENT TYPE (CIRCLE ONE):   1   2   3   4   5   6   7

NOTES:

	TIME:

SNACK 1 / LOCATION / NOTES:	
	TIME:
SNACK 2 / LOCATION / NOTES:	
	TIME:

LAST NIGHT'S SLEEP:

BEDTIME:	WAKETIME:

SLEEP QUALITY:

VITAMIN OR MEDICATION	REASON FOR TAKING	DOSAGE	DATE STARTED	COMMENTS/REACTIONS

DAILY H2O INTAKE (CROSS OUT A DROP FOR EVERY GLASS CONSUMED)

8 OZ.   8 OZ.   8 OZ.   8 OZ.   8 OZ.   8 OZ.   8 OZ.   8 OZ.   8 OZ.   8 OZ.

ADDITIONAL NOTES:

DATE: ....

MEAL 1 / LOCATION:	MOOD / SIGNS / SYMPTOMS / REACTIONS:
TIME:	

BOWEL MOVEMENT TYPE (CIRCLE ONE):	1	2	3	4	5	6	7

NOTES:

	TIME:

MEAL 2 / LOCATION:	MOOD / SIGNS / SYMPTOMS / REACTIONS:
TIME:	

BOWEL MOVEMENT TYPE (CIRCLE ONE):	1	2	3	4	5	6	7

NOTES:

	TIME:

MEAL 3 / LOCATION:	MOOD / SIGNS / SYMPTOMS / REACTIONS:
TIME:	

BOWEL MOVEMENT TYPE (CIRCLE ONE):	1	2	3	4	5	6	7

NOTES:

	TIME:

SNACK 1 / LOCATION / NOTES:	
	TIME:

SNACK 2 / LOCATION / NOTES:	
	TIME:

LAST NIGHT'S SLEEP:

BEDTIME:	WAKETIME:

SLEEP QUALITY:

VITAMIN OR MEDICATION	REASON FOR TAKING	DOSAGE	DATE STARTED	COMMENTS/REACTIONS

DAILY H2O INTAKE (CROSS OUT A DROP FOR EVERY GLASS CONSUMED)

8 OZ.   8 OZ.   8 OZ.   8 OZ.   8 OZ.   8 OZ.   8 OZ.   8 OZ.   8 OZ.   8 OZ.

ADDITIONAL NOTES:

DATE: ....

MEAL 1 / LOCATION:	MOOD / SIGNS / SYMPTOMS / REACTIONS:
TIME:	

BOWEL MOVEMENT TYPE (CIRCLE ONE):	1	2	3	4	5	6	7

NOTES:

TIME:

MEAL 2 / LOCATION:	MOOD / SIGNS / SYMPTOMS / REACTIONS:
TIME:	

BOWEL MOVEMENT TYPE (CIRCLE ONE):	1	2	3	4	5	6	7

NOTES:

TIME:

MEAL 3 / LOCATION:	MOOD / SIGNS / SYMPTOMS / REACTIONS:
TIME:	

BOWEL MOVEMENT TYPE (CIRCLE ONE):	1	2	3	4	5	6	7

NOTES:

TIME:

SNACK 1 / LOCATION / NOTES:	
	TIME:
SNACK 2 / LOCATION / NOTES:	
	TIME:

LAST NIGHT'S SLEEP:	
BEDTIME:	WAKETIME:
SLEEP QUALITY:	

VITAMIN OR MEDICATION	REASON FOR TAKING	DOSAGE	DATE STARTED	COMMENTS/REACTIONS

DAILY H2O INTAKE (CROSS OUT A DROP FOR EVERY GLASS CONSUMED)

8 OZ.   8 OZ.   8 OZ.   8 OZ.   8 OZ.   8 OZ.   8 OZ.   8 OZ.   8 OZ.   8 OZ.

ADDITIONAL NOTES:

DATE: ....

MEAL 1 / LOCATION:	MOOD / SIGNS / SYMPTOMS / REACTIONS:
TIME:	

BOWEL MOVEMENT TYPE (CIRCLE ONE):   1   2   3   4   5   6   7

NOTES:

	TIME:

MEAL 2 / LOCATION:	MOOD / SIGNS / SYMPTOMS / REACTIONS:
TIME:	

BOWEL MOVEMENT TYPE (CIRCLE ONE):   1   2   3   4   5   6   7

NOTES:

	TIME:

MEAL 3 / LOCATION:	MOOD / SIGNS / SYMPTOMS / REACTIONS:
TIME:	

BOWEL MOVEMENT TYPE (CIRCLE ONE):   1   2   3   4   5   6   7

NOTES:

	TIME:

SNACK 1 / LOCATION / NOTES:

	TIME:

SNACK 2 / LOCATION / NOTES:

	TIME:

LAST NIGHT'S SLEEP:

BEDTIME:	WAKETIME:

SLEEP QUALITY:

VITAMIN OR MEDICATION	REASON FOR TAKING	DOSAGE	DATE STARTED	COMMENTS/REACTIONS

DAILY H2O INTAKE (CROSS OUT A DROP FOR EVERY GLASS CONSUMED)

8 OZ.   8 OZ.   8 OZ.   8 OZ.   8 OZ.   8 OZ.   8 OZ.   8 OZ.   8 OZ.   8 OZ.

ADDITIONAL NOTES:

DATE: ....

MEAL 1 / LOCATION:	MOOD / SIGNS / SYMPTOMS / REACTIONS:
TIME:	
BOWEL MOVEMENT TYPE (CIRCLE ONE):　　1　　2　　3　　4　　5　　6　　7	
NOTES:	
	TIME:

MEAL 2 / LOCATION:	MOOD / SIGNS / SYMPTOMS / REACTIONS:
TIME:	
BOWEL MOVEMENT TYPE (CIRCLE ONE):　　1　　2　　3　　4　　5　　6　　7	
NOTES:	
	TIME:

MEAL 3 / LOCATION:	MOOD / SIGNS / SYMPTOMS / REACTIONS:
TIME:	
BOWEL MOVEMENT TYPE (CIRCLE ONE):　　1　　2　　3　　4　　5　　6　　7	
NOTES:	
	TIME:

SNACK 1 / LOCATION / NOTES:	
	TIME:
SNACK 2 / LOCATION / NOTES:	
	TIME:

LAST NIGHT'S SLEEP:

BEDTIME:	WAKETIME:

SLEEP QUALITY:

VITAMIN OR MEDICATION	REASON FOR TAKING	DOSAGE	DATE STARTED	COMMENTS/REACTIONS

DAILY H2O INTAKE (CROSS OUT A DROP FOR EVERY GLASS CONSUMED)

8 OZ. 8 OZ. 8 OZ. 8 OZ. 8 OZ. 8 OZ. 8 OZ. 8 OZ. 8 OZ. 8 OZ.

ADDITIONAL NOTES:

DATE: ....

MEAL 1 / LOCATION:	MOOD / SIGNS / SYMPTOMS / REACTIONS:
TIME:	

BOWEL MOVEMENT TYPE (CIRCLE ONE):	1	2	3	4	5	6	7

NOTES:

	TIME:

MEAL 2 / LOCATION:	MOOD / SIGNS / SYMPTOMS / REACTIONS:
TIME:	

BOWEL MOVEMENT TYPE (CIRCLE ONE):	1	2	3	4	5	6	7

NOTES:

	TIME:

MEAL 3 / LOCATION:	MOOD / SIGNS / SYMPTOMS / REACTIONS:
TIME:	

BOWEL MOVEMENT TYPE (CIRCLE ONE):	1	2	3	4	5	6	7

NOTES:

	TIME:

SNACK 1 / LOCATION / NOTES:	
	TIME:

SNACK 2 / LOCATION / NOTES:	
	TIME:

LAST NIGHT'S SLEEP:

BEDTIME:	WAKETIME:

SLEEP QUALITY:

VITAMIN OR MEDICATION	REASON FOR TAKING	DOSAGE	DATE STARTED	COMMENTS/REACTIONS

DAILY H2O INTAKE (CROSS OUT A DROP FOR EVERY GLASS CONSUMED)

8 OZ. 8 OZ. 8 OZ. 8 OZ. 8 OZ. 8 OZ. 8 OZ. 8 OZ. 8 OZ. 8 OZ.

ADDITIONAL NOTES:

DATE: ....

MEAL 1 / LOCATION:	MOOD / SIGNS / SYMPTOMS / REACTIONS:
TIME:	

BOWEL MOVEMENT TYPE (CIRCLE ONE):   1   2   3   4   5   6   7

NOTES:

	TIME:

MEAL 2 / LOCATION:	MOOD / SIGNS / SYMPTOMS / REACTIONS:
TIME:	

BOWEL MOVEMENT TYPE (CIRCLE ONE):   1   2   3   4   5   6   7

NOTES:

	TIME:

MEAL 3 / LOCATION:	MOOD / SIGNS / SYMPTOMS / REACTIONS:
TIME:	

BOWEL MOVEMENT TYPE (CIRCLE ONE):   1   2   3   4   5   6   7

NOTES:

	TIME:

SNACK 1 / LOCATION / NOTES:	
	TIME:

SNACK 2 / LOCATION / NOTES:	
	TIME:

LAST NIGHT'S SLEEP:

BEDTIME:	WAKETIME:

SLEEP QUALITY:

VITAMIN OR MEDICATION	REASON FOR TAKING	DOSAGE	DATE STARTED	COMMENTS/REACTIONS

DAILY H2O INTAKE (CROSS OUT A DROP FOR EVERY GLASS CONSUMED)

8 OZ.   8 OZ.   8 OZ.   8 OZ.   8 OZ.   8 OZ.   8 OZ.   8 OZ.   8 OZ.   8 OZ.

ADDITIONAL NOTES:

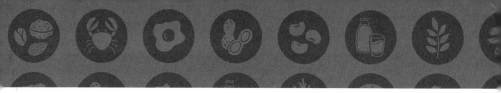

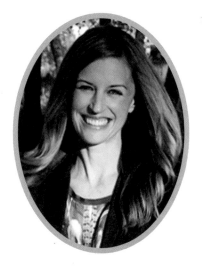

About the Author:

Molly Brennand is a Functional Nutrition and Lifestyle Practitioner and Holistic Health Coach based in Santa Fe, New Mexico. She is a graduate of the Institute for Integrative Nutrition and holds certifications from the Functional Nutrition Alliance in Full Body Systems and the Functional Nutrition and Lifestyle Practitioner program. Molly specializes in nutrition and lifestyle coaching for kids and adults navigating the complexities of chronic illness. She is most passionate about using food as medicine to support and empower individuals dealing with autism spectrum disorder, learning differences, sensory integration, and behavioral challenges. Molly offers both private and group coaching and is available for consultation at www.mollybrennand.com.